ESSENTIAL OHSAWA

ESSENTIAL OHSAWA

FROM FOOD TO HEALTH, HAPPINESS TO FREEDOM

GEORGE OHSAWA

Edited By Carl Ferré

Avery Publishing Group

Garden City Park, New York

By George Ohsawa
Art of Peace
Essential Ohsawa
Gandhi, the Eternal Youth
Macrobiotics, An Invitation to Health and Happiness
Macrobiotics, the Way of Healing
Order of the Universe
Philosophy of Oriental Medicine
Unique Principle
You Are All Sanpaku
Zen Macrobiotics

First Edition	1994
Second Printing	2002

Copyright © 1994 by George Ohsawa Macrobiotic Foundation
PO Box 3998, Chico, CA 95927-3998
800-232-2372, 530-566-9765, fax 530-5669768
Email: foundation@gomf.macrobiotic.net or gomf@earthlink.net

Cover design by Bill Gonzalez

Library of Congress Catalog Card Number: 93-46028
ISBN: 0-918860-57-1

Printed in the United States of America

CONTENTS

To George and Lima Ohsawa
who taught us to elevate our thoughts to the highest levels,
to explore the dimensions of infinite freedom,
and to live a life of complete health and eternal happiness.

FOREWORD

Like Lao-tsu, Confucius, and the prophets of the Old Testament, George Ohsawa envisioned a new era for humanity: an era of health, peace, and freedom for everyone. Being a man of thought *and* action, theory *and* practice, justice *and* love, George Ohsawa dedicated his life to the actual realization of health and peace. In other words, he did more than simply envision a new world; he was a citizen of that world and invited all of us to join him. In order for everyone to reach that destination, he offered a universal compass—in the form of the Unifying Principle—and a valid passport—in the form of a macrobiotic way of life.

With crystal-clear insight, Ohsawa revived, revitalized, and reinterpreted humanity's universal, traditional cosmology. He made it new, fresh, and accessible to everyone, using any and every opportunity to reveal its simplicity, practicality, and relevance. He applied this cosmology again and again on a practical level to show us how to change sickness into health, difficulty into ease, war into peace, and unhappiness into happiness.

As a person of endless compassion, Ohsawa undertook the challenge of sharing this universal treasure with everyone. He offered hope to people around the world and helped change the direction of civilization itself. For this reason, Ohsawa's appeal transcends time and place. People in all corners of the globe continue to be inspired by his vision, and also by his life story. As you will discover in the pages of *Essential Ohsawa*, the man is just as fascinating as the message. In fact, the two are inseparable.

Ohsawa appeared at a critical time in history: a time when the technological and industrial revolution threatened to alienate humanity from nature and from itself; when East and West clashed in a life-or-death struggle; when the destruction of the environment assumed global proportions; when the possibility of nuclear warfare threatened all life on Earth; and when the biological, psychological, and spiritual degeneration of humanity spread like wildfire across the planet. However, like the first rays of the morning sun appearing in the darkness, George Ohsawa's philosophy of natural living appeared as a necessary and refreshing antidote to these destructive trends. Contained in this philosophy—so succinctly presented in the following pages—are many ideas that are now commonly expressed. For example:

- Ohsawa's teachings about respect for nature and ecological living are the same as those of today's worldwide environmental movement, including the call to adopt grain- and vegetable-based diets to reverse environmental destruction. Moreover, Ohsawa's thinking on the economic justice of diet has been echoed in books such as *Diet for a Small Planet, Diet for a New America,* and others in which grain-, vegetable-, and soybean-based diets have been advocated as a solution to world hunger and a fundamental means for preserving scarce natural resources, including tropical rain forests.

- Ohsawa's emphasis on whole natural foods and his teaching that one's body and the soil are united in a very real way can now be heard in the organic, natural food, and natural farming movements. The use of pesticides and other chemicals in the production of food is now recognized as a threat to both personal and planetary health, and there is a call for a return to organic methods. Natural and organic foods are no longer restricted to specialized retail stores but are appearing with increasing frequency on supermarket shelves.

- Ohsawa's belief in the superiority of plant-based diets is now shared by medical scientists and researchers around the globe. This belief is being expressed in official reports, such as the landmark *Dietary Goals for the United States*, issued by the United States government in 1977. Population studies, such as the China Health Study, point to far lower rates of heart disease, cancer, diabetes, and other chronic diseases among people consuming grain- and vegetable-based diets.

- Ohsawa's introduction of Far Eastern and other traditional healing modalities—including acupuncture, moxibustion, herbal medicine, meditation, visualization, and other mind/body approaches—provided fertile soil for the growth of the holistic, alternative, and natural health movements, and for growing public acceptance of these approaches. In recent surveys, one-third of all Americans were found to be using alternative healing appproaches, including macrobiotics. Many physicians, other health-care providers, and the United States National Institutes of Health (NIH) are studying and investigating alternative medicine. Ohsawa's dream of a synthesis of Eastern and Western medicine may occur sooner than we think.

- Ohsawa's teaching that eating a balanced diet of whole natural foods can help reverse chronic and acute illness, confirmed by over fifty years of experience, is now being taken seriously by medical science. On the biochemical front, researchers are discovering numerous compounds in grains, beans, sea vegetables, miso, and fresh vegetables that inhibit the growth of cancerous tumors. On the clinical front, studies such as those conducted by Dr. Dean Ornish, in which a grain- and vegetable-based diet was found to reverse long-standing coronary blockage, a leading cause of heart attack and stroke, confirm Ohsawa's faith in the healing power of one's own body, given the right nourishment.

  The increasing popularity of macrobiotics among persons with cancer along with the publication of documented stories of cancer recovery has led NIH to approve an official study of macrobiotics and cancer. In the near future, a naturally balanced diet along the lines of macrobiotics may become a primary component of the modern health-care system. In addition, Ohsawa's teaching about personal responsibility for health is gaining increasing acceptance in the fields of public health and preventive medicine.

- Ohsawa's pioneering discoveries in atomic transmutation along with his application of yin and yang in the world of chemistry and physics helped pave the way for the appearance of an entirely new school of scientific thought. In this new school, all things are seen as interrelated, not separate, and the Cartesian division between mind and body, observer and observed, and humanity and nature is being replaced by a more holistic and unifying paradigm.

- Ohsawa's vision of a planetary civilization united by a common dream of health, peace, respect for nature, and an intuitive awareness of our origin and destiny as human beings, is steadily being realized as his ideas continue to spread across national, racial, ideological, and geographic boundaries. From Sydney to St. Petersburg, Boston to Buenos Aires, Colorado to the Congo, Oroville to Osaka, a growing number of people are pursuing Ohsawa's ideas.

Essential Ohsawa should do much to further Ohsawa's vision. I have often dreamed about a book such as this during my years as a teacher of macrobiotics at the Kushi Institute in the Berkshires and throughout the world. I thank Herman and Cornellia Aihara, Carl Ferré, and the staff of the George Ohsawa Macrobiotic Foundation for their patient effort in producing *Essential Ohsawa*. I also thank Rudy Shur of Avery Publishing Group for inspiring the Foundation to undertake this worthwhile project. This book is indeed a treasure.

I hope you enjoy Ohsawa and accept his smiling invitation to a new world of health, happiness, and infinite adventure.

Edward Esko

PREFACE

For many years, Herman and Cornellia Aihara, founders of the George Ohsawa Macrobiotic Foundation and Vega Study Center, and I had dreamed of producing a multi-volume series containing all of Ohsawa's books in order to make his thinking more accessible to people. This project had not materialized partly due to the enormity of the task but also because many of the books are restatements of the same thing: An explanation of the Order of the Universe and its practical application to natural living.

The idea for *Essential Ohsawa* was born a few years ago at the Vega Study Center in Northern California during a meeting with Rudy Shur of Avery Publishing Group. Rudy had come to meet with Herman and Cornellia regarding publication of their book *Natural Healing From Head to Toe*. After discussing the Aiharas' work, Rudy asked if we'd be interested in having Avery publish a book of Ohsawa's writings containing a definitive statement of the most salient aspects of Ohsawa's beliefs. Thus, Rudy's idea crystallized our project to a manageable size and was met with great enthusiasm.

First, all of Ohsawa's works available in English were copied, organized by subject, and retyped. Then began the fascinating task of distilling a file cabinet full of material into one cohesive book. During the process, it became obvious that this book should contain the underlying principles of Ohsawa's ideas and writings along with a sampling of the great variety of subjects about which he wrote. These subjects range from science to religion and from guidelines for daily living to matters of the spirit and one's ultimate dreams. Thus, the book is arranged into three parts: Foundations of the Body, Principles of the Mind, and Dreams of the Spirit.

Part One contains Ohsawa's thinking on diet, health, and curing disease. He truly believed that simple, natural eating and drinking lead to health. This method had worked for him—acutally, it had saved his life—and he saw many thousands of people helped by it during his lifetime. However, Ohsawa didn't want people to blindly follow any dietary or health practice, including his own; he wanted people to have a thorough understanding of the principles behind it. As he wrote, "Any art, practice, or technique is quite dangerous if it has no firm, theoretical foundation."

The foundations of Ohsawa's dietary practice are described in Part Two, which includes his ideas on increasing one's judging ability and on education, yin-yang theory, and the origins of Far Eastern philosophy. Ohsawa also believed, as he wrote, "Any theory, be it scientific, religious, or philosophical, is quite useless if it is too difficult to understand or impractical for daily living." His own theories are understandable with minimal effort and are very practical.

The real power of Ohsawa's thought, and some of his most inspiring writing, is contained in Part Three. Here, his thinking on the ultimate human desires of happiness, peace, and freedom are presented. Ohsawa taught that while a healthy body and mind can bring one partial happiness, the greatest happiness is achieved in giving to others. Such happiness leads to infinite freedom and eternal peace.

The postmatter contains a brief End Note by me, a chronology of the events in Ohsawa's life by Herman Aihara, and a list of the writings of Ohsawa compiled by Herman and me.

The writings included in this book have been taken from many works and edited to make a unified presentation. Those who have read Ohsawa's original works, or those who will do so, should be aware of decisions made in the editing process.

Ohsawa wrote in Japanese, French, and English for a great variety of audiences. He used language to appeal to the Japanese before, during, and after World War II; to the French in the 1950s; and to the Americans in the early 1960s. Ohsawa spent many years in France and the United States and loved the West. However, his writings for the Japanese before and during the war had to be anti-West in order to be read or even published. Most of this anti-West tone has been omitted from this book.

His writing on diet was written with the French in mind. Ohsawa had observed that no matter how limited he made his dietary suggestions, the French always cheated and ate a broader range of foods. Thus, he made a dietary suggestion of brown rice, gomashio (sesame salt), and a little bancha tea only. This diet became known as diet number seven and was to be used for short times as with a fast. When this diet was brought to the United States, however, Americans were able to follow it without cheating and for long and, at times, dangerous periods of time. However, much of Ohsawa's writing on diet is consistent with today's macrobiotic practice, and it is this writing that has been included here.

Ohsawa liked to shock people in order to move them to action. Thus, his writing can be extreme at times. While enough of this more extreme writing has been included for flavor, much of it has been omitted because it serves no useful purpose in understanding Ohsawa's philosophy in this day and age. If you want full-strength Ohsawa, you may wish to read the complete originals.

Ohsawa wrote mostly at a time when the terms "man" or "mankind" were commonly used in reference to both men and women. Rather than update this, the language has been left in its original form and is not intended to be exclusionary in any way.

Most of Ohsawa's books available in English were translated from Japanese or from Ohsawa's French. It is difficult to convey the meanings exactly, and to compound the difficulty, all of Ohsawa's works available in English, including those written in English, had previously been edited by many people. Thus, the writing style varies slightly from section to section. However, terms that have been used in different ways in the various writings have been changed in this book so that their usage is consistent.

For example, Ohsawa used both the term "Unifying Principle" and the term "Unique Principle" to describe his philosophy. Even though the ideas are quite unique and Ohsawa used "Unique Principle" for its shock value, "Unifying Principle" has been chosen because it better conveys Ohsawa's message of the unification of all things.

It is rare in this day of specialists to find a person with such a broad understanding of so many fields. Ohsawa was a philosopher in the original sense of the word—one who studies the principles that cause, control, and explain facts, events, and life itself. We perceive of a philosopher as a person sitting at a desk lost in books most of his or her life. However, Ohsawa was a philosopher of action. He was the greatest of adventurers, travelling the world, conducting endless experiments on himself, and spending time in jail for his beliefs.

Photos and remembrances of Ohsawa by those who knew him personally have been included to help show his human side. If you are fortunate enough to know any of the authors of these remembrances, take the opportunity to ask them about Ohsawa. Watch their faces light up, their voices fill with enthusiasm, and their spirits be uplifted once again when they remember the man who helped give the very meaning of life to so many.

Carl Ferré

ESSENTIAL
OHSAWA

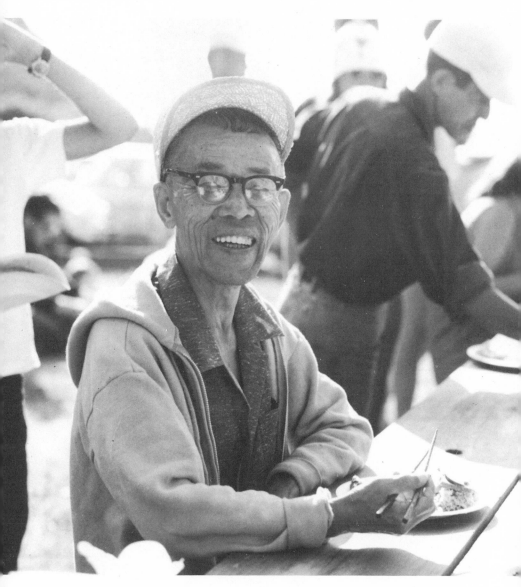

George Ohsawa picnicking at Big Sur, 1963. Herman Aihara is seen in background, wearing a cap

INTRODUCTION

According to the Japanese police during World War II, George
Ohsawa was a persistent peace activist; according to some American medical doctors, he was a dangerous dietitian; according to
Japanese media reporters, he was a fortuneteller who had pre-
dicted the deaths of Gandhi and Kennedy; according to American
media reports, he was an occult leader who enticed some young
people to become hippies; and according to many people throughout the world, he was a profound healer of body and soul. So just
who is George Ohsawa?

George Ohsawa (Yukizaku Sakurazawa, 1893–1966) is recognized as the founder of macrobiotic principles and lifestyle practices.
However, he had so many interests in life and did so much in a short
time that it is difficult to describe him in such a brief way. His words,
actions, and influence spread over the entire world, and yet every
word we say about him covers merely a part of him. At the very least,
he was a scholar, healer, businessman, educator, and poet.

But most of all, he was a Far Eastern philosopher who taught
his version of the ancient Chinese philosophy of yin and yang.
When he was in France, he first applied his philosophy to physical
science. Later, he worked to apply it to many areas such as nutrition, diet, medicine, chemistry, ethics, religion, education, and
business, as well as lifestyle. Ohsawa also collected many of the
great thoughts from East and West, from ancient to modern, and

applied them to various aspects of living. His interpretations, based on the Unifying Principle of yin and yang, were devised to guide people in a practical way toward health and happiness.

On the one hand, Ohsawa was a man of love, kindness, and gentleness who wanted to help unhappy, sick, and weak people. Therefore, he established both a hospital in which he counselled almost one hundred people every day and night and a study center where any unhappy person could study with him without charge and follow his dietary recommendations and philosophy. I was fortunate to be one of the many young people he educated at his center. Every morning between 2:00 and 6:00, he wrote letters to students who had left his center, no matter where they were in the world. Such letters amounted to thousands of pages a year. He did this because he was a man of caring and love.

On the other hand, Ohsawa's criticism of others was fierce and persistent, like a sword. His criticism was so severe at times that students were afraid to be near him. This part of his character made his educational discipline very severe, but his criticism was always tempered by his loving and caring side. For example, Ohsawa allowed mistakes at his study center if the mistakes were admitted. However, he didn't allow anyone to make excuses for mistakes. If someone made an excuse for a mistake, Ohsawa scolded and pinpointed every reason that the person must take sole responsibility for the mistake until the mistake was admitted from the heart. In this way, no one ever made the same mistake again. Thus, he was a wonderful educator. However, many students left his school because of his scolding.

Ohsawa's favorite motto was "Non Credo" ("don't believe"), always see for yourself. For him, unhappiness was the result of poor thinking ability. He gave students two to three questions every day and expected answers or reports the next morning. He told us not to be imitators. If students answered his questions using someone else's idea or writing, he gave them a minus mark, even if it was the right answer. He was happier if the answer was a student's own thinking, even if it was wrong. This is because Ohsawa was not interested in whether we had the factual knowledge to answer his questions, rather he wanted us to answer with our infinite yin and yang thinking. Yin and yang thinking is determining cold or hot, left or right, expanded or contracted, and so on, and can be used at any time and in every circumstance. Such yin and yang thinking is more intuitive and is what Ohsawa was interested in teaching instead of factual knowledge.

Ohsawa also taught us always to accept new challenges and more difficulties. According to him, solving difficulties makes one most joyous and happy. Easily attained or externally supplied joy and happiness are not lasting or deep. He taught us to change sickness to health, sadness to joy, poverty to wealth, enemies to friends. If you are able to do this once, do it twice, and then three times. Then you will understand that changing unhappiness to happiness is the *real* happiness and joy. Still, this happiness is limited in this finite world.

By understanding our mental and physiological limitations, we enter the infinite, spiritual world where our thinking is completely free. This is the entrance to the greatest happiness. For this, Ohsawa recommended understanding beyond yin and yang thinking to what he called "the Order of the Universe." Yin and yang exist in the antagonistic, finite world, but in the infinite, unified world, there is nothing, not even yin and yang. Thus, the main emphasis of his teaching was on understanding the Order of the Universe and identifying your place in this order. "Who are you?" is the question Ohsawa asked students. Anyone who completely understood and answered this question, instantly cured any sickness. In my opinion, there were very few students who reached such an understanding. Some understood within one month. Others never understood and gave up macrobiotics, even after many years of following Ohsawa.

As requested of his students, Ohsawa himself was an eternal student and researcher of truth. He was driven by a passion for finding the origin of all things—the very beginnings of life itself. His relentless searching took him to many lands and through the literature of all the major thinkers and religions. He was a fast reader and every month wrote more than ten opinions or reports on the books or magazines he had read. His reports were so thorough, unique, and interesting that I learned more from his writings than from the originals. He read and subsequently talked and wrote about a great variety of subjects such as anthropology, biology, chemistry, economics, diet, education, history, industry, Japan, macrobiotics, medicine, nutrition, philosophy, physics, politics, the West, and, of course, yin and yang.

There is no doubt that Ohsawa's search began with events in his childhood. As Ohsawa himself relates it:

> I saw the deaths of my thirty-year-old mother and my younger sister and brother occur as a direct consequence of the introduction of Western foods and medicine into their lives. Then came my turn. Being a very poor orphan of nine, I fortunately could not continue the new Westernized food and medicine for financial reasons. Even so, I was dying at sixteen from the large quantities of chemically-refined sugar and sweets that I continued to use. At eighteen, I rediscovered the Far Eastern medicine with its solid basis in a cosmological philosophy. It cured me completely.

Once he discovered that eating a simple, natural diet can lead to health, Ohsawa became a strong proponent of and hard worker for Shoku-Yo Kai, an association in Japan that was carrying on the work of Sagen Ishizuka. Ishizuka had taught that one's health depends on a proper balance of sodium and potassium salts, and his dietary regime of whole brown rice, vegetables, salt, and oil became the basis of a macrobiotic dietary approach. After years of study and refinement, Ohsawa added the theoretical foundation of yin and yang philosophy and began to use the term "macrobiotic" to describe his approach to life and health. Once Ohsawa's macrobiotic organization was firmly established in Japan, Ohsawa went to France to present to the Western world the Unifying Principle of yin and yang and its application to a macrobiotic diet.

During his stay in Paris, while enduring the poorest of living conditions, he was busy studying Western science at the Sorbonne Institute, publishing original works and French translations of Japanese books, and introducing to the West aspects of Far Eastern culture such as acupuncture, judo, flower arrangement, and haiku. When Ohsawa returned to Japan, he introduced elements of Western culture to the East, translating important French and English works into Japanese.

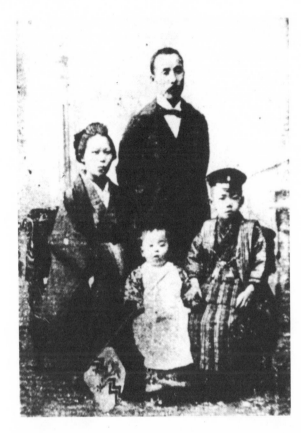

*George Ohsawa
as a child (right)
with his parents
and younger
brother, 1901.*

Ohsawa's view of the world encompassed both East and West, and he tried to help each understand the other for the betterment of all. When Ohsawa read the title *The Great Ideas: A Syntopicon of Great Books of the World*, edited by Mortimer J. Adler, he immediately wrote the publisher explaining that the title was misleading because it did not include any ideas or books of the East. Upon hearing this critique, the publisher changed the title to *The Great Ideas: A Syntopicon of Great Books of the Western World*.

It was the climate of impending war in Japan that led to Ohsawa's return to his native land. He devoted his life just as passionately to stopping World War II as he had to furthering macrobiotic ideas. Because he published many antiwar books and magazine articles, Ohsawa was constantly sought by the military police and was jailed many times. He was sentenced to death twice because of his antiwar activities but managed to survive until General MacArthur released him after Japan surrendered in 1945. He remained a world peace activist for the rest of his life.

At the age of sixty, he left Japan on a world lecture trip to teach macrobiotic principles, diet, and way of life. This trip created macrobiotic movements all over the world. It was like a typhoon, and Ohsawa was the eye of the typhoon. Everywhere he went, a macrobiotic movement sprouted. While there were students who preceded him to many countries, it was Ohsawa's visits that provided the spark for the movement. Hundreds of thousands of people were helped and inspired as a direct result of his tireless work.

Ohsawa's profound effect on people can be seen in the number of his students still actively teaching macrobiotics. In the United States, Cornellia Aihara and I operate the George Ohsawa Macrobiotic Foundation and Vega Study Center in Northern California. Michio and Aveline Kushi founded and teach at the Kushi Institute in Western Massachusetts and travel extensively throughout the world spreading macrobiotics. Junsei and Kazuko Yamazaki are actively teaching in Northern California; Shizuko Yamamoto in New York City; Cecile Levin in Los Angeles; Michel Matsuda in North Carolina; and many others continue to teach and/or practice the way of life they learned directly from Ohsawa some thirty or more years ago.

And it is no different throughout the world. Ohsawa's philosophy is taught in France by Francoise Rivière and Renè Levy, in Belgium by Clim Yoshimi, in Brazil by Tomio Kikuchi, and in Vietnam, India, and a host of other countries by Ohsawa's former students. The largest number of former students is in Japan, and the activities there continue to flourish under the able guidance of Lima Ohsawa at the age of ninety-four.

The basic foundations of Ohsawa's macrobiotic philosophy have not changed, but the depth of people's understanding has diminished somewhat. Newer students seem interested only in re-establishing their physical health and use only one small application of the Unifying Principle of yin and yang—namely, a macrobiotic diet—for this purpose. All around me, I hear people saying, "The macrobiotic diet this . . ." and "the macrobiotic diet that. . . ." It's as if they can't see the beauty of the forest because the trees are in the way. You can literally change your life, become free from fear, elevate your consciousness, and live with total joy by using Ohsawa's method. However, as Ohsawa said many times, "I can only give you the keys, you must unlock the door. There are many doors, you must decide which one to open."

However, times have changed, people have changed, and the macrobiotic approach also has had to change. Just as Ohsawa changed his strategy many times during his life, I have no doubt that if he were alive today, he would change his presentation to meet the challenges of today's world with the same enthusiasm and dedication that he showed throughout his life.

Although Ohsawa changed his activities due to political and other reasons, his goal was always the same: To educate people and world leaders about his concepts of the Unifying Principle and the Order of the Universe and the importance of a macrobiotic understanding and diet in creating a world of peace and happiness. The essence of this macrobiotic philosophy is that everyone is free to change from unhealthy slaves of money and medicine to healthy and happy individuals who can think for themselves.

Thus, if you want to solve any problem, including the lack of world peace, you must begin with yourself. By eating and drinking naturally and in an orderly manner through an application of the yin and yang philosophy, you can establish and maintain your health. True health leads to real happiness, and a peaceful society can only be built by a group of truly happy individuals. Through daily practice, dedication, and will power, anything—including absolute happiness, eternal peace, and infinite freedom—can be achieved.

These words and ideas persist even though George Ohsawa died on April 24, 1966, at the age of seventy-three. According to Dr. Ushio, a physician who was also macrobiotic, the cause of death was arterial thrombosis. Nobody really knows why Ohsawa developed this condition. In my opinion, it was his lack of sleep. He used to say that sleep was a waste of time and that he didn't need to sleep. He tried to prove it. Therefore, he was sleep-deprived most of his life. He wanted to make other people happy, and he gave himself no time to relax or to seek amusement or comfort. He devoted the whole of his life to teaching macrobiotics to the entire world. He wrote over three hundred books and lectured over five thousand times in Japan, England, France, Belgium, Germany, America, Africa, India, and Vietnam. He was sentenced to death twice. He was tortured many times by the military police in Japan during World War II. I do not know how many times he was jailed. He had little or no money most of his life. None of these hardships ever changed his decision to teach macrobiotics. He always pushed himself to the limit.

A few years ago, I read a report about an old Russian man still living at the age of one hundred sixty-three. He had never left his native land nor made friends outside of his village. Ohsawa also could have lived for more than one hundred years if he had not pushed himself so strongly. However, Ohsawa just could not live a quiet, homebound life like the old Russian. The length of one's life should be measured by the height of happiness achieved, the number of friends made, and their influence on others even after death. From this point of view, Ohsawa has lived a thousand years or more. Jesus Christ and Lao-tsu are similar examples. Their lives were not so long compared to the old Russian man's, but they are still living in us. I hope an understanding of Ohsawa's philosophy will extend your life and happiness to the fullest extent possible.

Herman Aihara

Part One

FOUNDATIONS
OF THE BODY

Let us make our bodies healthy with righteous food.
We can thus enter into the miracles of the universe
and enjoy a profound eternal life.

George Ohsawa
Macrobiotic Guidebook for Living

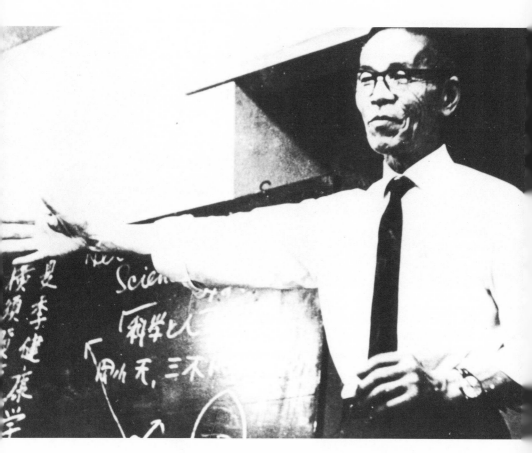

George Ohsawa lecturing in Japan, 1965.

1

NATURAL EATING AND DRINKING

NATURAL FOODS

Leaves of grass—green, simple, beautiful, natural—shapes endless in variety yet never strange, unfamiliar, or artificial. . . .

No one can duplicate this naturalness. We can analyze its parts, imitate its color or form; but its vitality, its physiological and chemical activity, its power to grow—all of this eludes us. Human understanding cannot encompass it.

There is no factory in existence that can remove carbon dioxide from the air, produce its own oxygen, and then change the whole thing into carbohydrate with the addition of a little sunshine. Yet this complex process occurs simply and with little effort in a blade of grass.

A tree—fifty or even seventy feet tall with roots that go deep into the earth; branches that reach out in every direction, that bow to the ground in the grip of a storm and then spring back to their former shape and position with the ceasing of the wind. Rain is its sweet bath, snow its wrap of ermine. No complaint or protest—it gratefully accepts both good and bad.

Seen at a distance in its totality, the tree that has stood for a hundred years or more is a thing of natural beauty. It is so simple. If we approach more closely, if we examine its detail under a microscope or analyze it chemically, we find a complex miracle forever beyond our comprehension.

The living human, God's natural product, has a deceptively simple exterior: two arms, two legs, a torso, a head. But examine them closely—what complexity! A hand consists of only one palm and five fingers, but its wonderful power has made history through an endless variety of acts, both virtuous and criminal. This seemingly elementary tool has produced all of civilization.

Biologists and anatomists have found what they have labelled heart, lungs, nerves, and intestines—small, quiet mechanisms covered by skin. The life that causes them to function, however, is a complexity that resists analysis.

And what of memory? We easily remember things that have happened thirty or forty years in the past and enjoy singing songs learned in childhood. What device can record, file away, and instantaneously replay memories from so long ago? Perhaps someone will eventually construct one but it will be far more complicated than our human function, just as the finest camera cannot compare with the complex simplicity of the human eye.

Human productivity always appears complex on its surface. A house, an airplane, a watch, a radio—each is a mass of detail that proves to be very simple upon close scrutiny.

Health or true life, a natural state of being for living things, is simple. It is soundless—no motor runs so quietly. When we attempt to discover and analyze all its details, however, we undertake the same impossibly useless task we faced in probing the mysteries of the blade of grass or the tree.

The apparent simplicity of nature that is revealed to be infinite complication itself requires only earth, sunshine, wind, and water for full existence. A man needs no more to be assured a joyous life.

In the morning, he awakens easily to find that he has visitors— a breeze that is the breath of God, sunshine that is the glance of the Mother of Life. He eats naturally—grains, seeds, leaves, roots, grasses in all forms. He adds a few grains of salt—a reminder of his briny origin. This and some clear spring water. Nothing more. How simple and uncomplicated a breakfast table.

Natural cuisine has the taste of the primitive, the flavor of *haiku* and the tea ceremony. Its final product is simplicity itself yet it holds infinite complexity within. It has the taste of nature. He who cannot distinguish it from that of the artificial, elaborate food found in restaurants and supermarkets will spend a sad life because he is caught in a web of artificiality. He will surely spoil his health and his life will end tragically.

Of late, many people have become enthusiastic about hiking, mountain-climbing, skiing, and camping. Most of them are trying to find or maintain health through some kind of contact with nature; they seek her out with a vengeance. Meanwhile, their rucksacks are bursting with chocolate, candy, wine, butter, canned goods, ham, sausage—all processed foods. It is hard for me to understand how they can devote themselves so energetically to the pursuit of Nature and still bring such unnatural foodstuffs into her presence. It is like working long hours to buy a plane ticket to Tokyo and then blindly boarding a plane that flies in the opposite direction.

Natural food is so very important because it is the condensation or crystallization of sunshine, air, and water—the source of life. Sunshine, air, and water are not too difficult to find in their original forms but the search for natural food involves problems.

Most of what we eat today comes to us from remote places; it grows in one season and we use it during another. It is consequently frozen and/or artificially preserved in order to be salable. Even those things that are produced in nearer places have been grown with chemical fertilizers and insecticides to protect them and stimulate growth. They are all unnatural foods.

All commercial fruits today are grown with strong insecticides and chemical fertilizers that are harmful to human beings and are inevitably poisonous. They are unnaturally cultivated products that are far removed from what nature intended as is indicated by their lack of flavor, their exaggerated size, and their excessive potassium content.

Commercially prepared cakes are no different. They are made with tropical sugar and chocolate that originate at a distance of many miles. They contain artificial coloring and preservatives that, while they do not kill a man instantaneously, will wear him away in time.

To eat such foods is to commit slow suicide. To produce them is to be guilty of slow murder.

Saints and wise men have long advised, "Return to nature." But because they have been so abstract and mystical about how this is achieved, it has been the rare individual who has succeeded in living by their words.

Some have tried forsaking the conveniences of the civilized world—cars, radios, telephones, steam heat—and have only changed the external, superficial part of their lives. Even if we live like our animal cousins—unshaven, unwashed, unclad, sleeping on a bed of pine needles with a blanket of leaves as our cover—nature eludes us.

Yet the method that makes a return to nature possible is so very simple. There is no other way than by making ourselves, our organisms, one with her. We must eat natural foods.

The world of life is governed by the law of God: *shin do fu ji*, meaning the body and the land are not two (separated or divided). Whoever ignores this suffers just punishment—sickness, deterioration, degeneration—because he cannot adapt to his surroundings. Neither individuals, nor races, nor man as a whole is exempt.

The healthy, happy man has understood that to live a joyful life, no matter where on this earth, he must first of all make himself one with his environment. He must eat, drink, and behave in a manner that does not alienate him from the orderly, simple truth of nature.

He must discover natural food—that which grows in his immediate area—uncontaminated by the imposed, artificial protection that science misguidedly offers through insecticides, pesticides, artificial fertilizers, preservatives, and additives.

If we want to live in this world—so joyful and yet so severe because it offers no way out of the punishment that is dealt to those who swim against the current of life, the orderliness of the universe—we must look to and never forget nature.

In our material world, two viewpoints exist side by side, again reminding us that yin and yang are ever present everywhere.

The mechanical, analytical, scientific viewpoint sees all things

My New Life

I first heard about macrobiotics at one of Ohsawa's seminars when I was thirty-five. Since the audience filled the auditorium, I couldn't see him personally; however, his talk was my big surprise. What he said was unbelievable news for me and I thought, "Someday I will be cured, even though I have been sickly my whole life!" In fact, I had visited six major hospitals in Tokyo to consult with doctors about my sicknesses. I was weak and had no appetite. Since I had no appetite, I couldn't eat even white rice.

As soon as I heard Ohsawa's lecture, I started a macrobiotic diet. I stopped eating my most favorite foods like sugar and fruits and began eating brown rice, which I have continued to eat for well over fifty years now. I joined Ohsawa's Macrobiotic Association and went there to buy foods, and he gave me a dietary list. That was my beginning in macrobiotics.

Since then, my life has completely changed. From being a fearful and frail traditional housewife, I became a woman who travelled the seven seas and cured thousands of sicknesses, including my husband's deadly sicknesses several times. That is a brief picture of my encounter with Ohsawa and my new life.

Lima Ohsawa
Wife of George Ohsawa

as separate—separated from themselves, separate from men. Not only are they apart from man in this sense, but they are created to be subservient to him, subject to his every whim.

With this as justification, men arrogantly impose themselves upon one another and their surroundings in a vain effort to find happiness, health, and peace. The end result is disease, tragedy, and war.

The spiritual viewpoint that originates in seventh heaven or infinity sees all things as being one. Nature is God; God is truth;

truth is the eternal order that simplifies infinite complexity to the greatest degree.

Everyone without exception has the right to know truth. For that very reason, truth has the responsibility to be uncomplicated—simple. For the same reason, the principle of life and health—macrobiotic eating and drinking, the nutritional path to longevity—is truth because it is so simple.

Health—not merely the absence of disease, but the dynamic balance that nature maintains so effortlessly—is the usual state of beings in the universe. It is natural and simple; it is identical with order; it cannot be produced artificially with machines or pills, science notwithstanding.

If health is natural, what could be more fitting and orderly than to achieve a state of well-being by following the simple way of nature? If you comprehend this, you are a poet. Your understanding of the consummate beauty of nature is such that your life itself becomes poetry. And all that you write is poetic without your having set out to make it so.

Intuitively, without material proof being necessary, we know that nature or God or the whole exists. Our spirit, our soul, our mind intuits or recognizes it by a method that is beyond logic, a way that is superlogical. In reality, intuition is the manifestation of wholeness itself.

Our human body is part of the whole. It owes its very existence to it. The whole is nature and whole nature is our spirit.

To know God, to recall nature, to acknowledge wholeness is the highest wisdom to which a human being can aspire. The highest form of discipline with which to achieve such wisdom is the macrobiotic way of living.

THE VEGETAL MOTHER

The first principles of nutrition are simple:

1. He who eats, exists.
2. He who eats can think, speak, act, love, hate, quarrel, attack another, kill himself, and marry.

3. He who does not eat can do nothing. He must of necessity disappear.

Neither Buddha nor Jesus could come and preach in this world without foods. No biological or even mental or social phenomena can appear in a foodless country. Like all other beings, man is a transformation of foods. But what are the foods? My first discovery in dietetics was that all our foods have a vegetal origin. They are produced from chlorophyll; thus, the animal cannot exist without the vegetal.

The human body cannot digest inorganic substances or manufacture from them proteins, carbohydrates, fats, vitamins, minerals, etc. The synthesizing and vitalizing of inorganic elements is a vegetal function. This process is called autotropism. Only the vegetable kingdom can perform this phenomenon. Vegetables absorb inorganic elements and convert them into organic foods, which are very complicated in their composition and construction. This is a veritable miracle produced by the interworking of the forces of nature.

The vegetal works continuously to produce leaves, grains, tubers, and fruits to feed the animals. The vegetal is mother to all animals. It is transformed into the animal by the process of digestion and assimilation. If, while walking under the green foliage in a forest, we feel a sensation of very agreeable quietness, it is because we are feeling a bit like a child kissed, caressed, and petted by his mother.

Each animal serves its purpose but we have no need to feed ourselves with meat or animal products, save for pleasure. Pleasure always has a limit. For instance, sugar (yin) eaten in excess is carcinogenic; too much animal protein (yang) results in thrombosis, cruelty, violence, etc.

Biologically speaking, we are children of the vegetal mother; we spring from the vegetal. Without vegetable life, no animal on the Earth would survive. We depend upon vegetal products. Our hemoglobin is derived from chlorophyll. All vegetal foods are virgin materials for the purpose of maintaining or constructing our body. Neither meat nor animal products are pure virgin material for us. We must eat vegetables and their direct products. This is the biological principle and fundamental law: Vegetables are the superior food.

PRINCIPAL FOOD

The strangest thing in the West, it would appear to me, is the total absence of the most fundamental concept for living, namely principal food. My most significant discovery in America, fully as important as the one made by Christopher Columbus, is that here the idea of a principal food has entirely disappeared. No professor or man of medicine nowadays seems to be aware of its great value.

The idea of principal food, the basis and significance of which is primarily biological and physiological, and only secondarily economical, geographical, and agricultural, is one of the most fundamental discoveries of man. It is fully as significant as the discovery of fire, which enabled man to create civilization (the union of religion, philosophy, science, and technology), and which determined the history of the evolution of food.

Of course, one can live by eating almost anything that pleases either the sensory, sentimental, intellectual, economical, moral, or ideological judgment. (The Stages of Judgment are explained beginning on page 73.) But there is a limit to such eating, namely unhappiness, which includes a variety of difficulties like illness, slavery, crime, and war.

At one time, the clearly distinguished concept of principal and secondary food enabled the people of the Far East to live a relatively happy, free, and peaceful life. This concept produced a diet of eating only the foods necessary for man.

What are the foods necessary for man? Good air, water, and sunshine are necessary for man to sustain life. Lacking one of them will lead to destruction of the human being. Therefore, these are the most important foods. Other foods that are necessary for man, such as whole grains, vegetables, beans, sea vegetables, and fish, are products or transformations of these three basic foods.

Furthermore, the proper foods for man are those that are traditionally eaten, locally grown, and seasonal in that particular location. In other words, the right foods for man agree with ecological law. Man, like any other living thing, is a product of nature, a biological creature. Therefore, he must observe biological and ecological laws, which tell us that soil produces vegetables and grasses, which in turn sustain the life of animals. Therefore, as the ancient Chinese believed: The soil and our body are inseparably related. The first macrobiotic principle, that our food must be locally grown and in season, is drawn from this relationship.

Table 1.1 on page 20 lists foods in various categories and from yin to yang. [An explanation of yin and yang can be found in Part Two, pages 105–130.] Only whole grains are meant to be used as principal foods. They can be eaten daily and at every meal. They form the foundation of a macrobiotic way of eating because they are a combination of both seed and fruit, are abundant on the Earth, and are a most economical, ecological, and nutritious food. Only a whole grain diet will solve the starvation problem due to overpopulation, because, for one reason, four thousand pounds of grain can be produced per acre, while only two hundred pounds of meat can be produced per acre.

All other food and drink listed, whether yin or yang, is to be used in smaller quantities, occasionally, and with care. For example, apple, although it is listed as the most yang fruit, cannot be safely eaten in the same quantity as whole brown rice. Even though apples are yang among fruits, the entire category of fruit is a very yin one as compared to the whole grains category.

The food and drink categories themselves, e.g. whole grains, vegetables, etc., are in an order that designates the quantity to be used (percentage of total food served) and the frequency with which they are used.

The foods to avoid are products of chemical fertilizer and sprays; synthetic or mass-produced foods; products of different localities and seasons; hot-house products; colored, preserved, bleached, or artificially sweetened products; and those containing chemicalized seasonings.

Whole Grains

Whole grains are always used as the basis for a meal. They are used

Table 1.1 Foods and Beverages*

[Listed within each category in order from yin (▼) to yang (▲)]

1. Whole Grains
- ▼Corn
- Rye
- Barley
- Oats
- Cracked wheat
- Wheat
- Millet
- ▲Rice (whole, brown)
- ▲▲Buckwheat

2. Vegetables
- ▼▼▼Eggplant
- Tomato
- Sweet potato
- Potato
- Shiitake mushroom
- Pimento
- Most beans
- Cucumber
- Asparagus
- Spinach
- Artichoke
- Bamboo sprout
- Mushroom
- ▼▼Green pea
- Celery
- Lentil
- ▼Purple cabbage
- Beet
- White cabbage
- ▲Dandelion (leaf and stem)
- Lettuce
- Endive
- Kale
- Radish
- Garlic
- Onion
- Parsley
- ▲▲Hokkaido pumpkin
- Carrot
- Coltsfoot
- Burdock
- Watercress
- Dandelion (root)
- ▲▲▲Jinenjo

3. Fish
- ▼Oyster
- Clam
- Octopus
- Eel
- Carp
- Moule
- Halibut
- Lobster
- Trout
- Sole
- ▲Salmon
- Shrimp
- Herring
- Sardine
- Red snapper (tai)
- ▲▲Caviar

4. Animal Products
- ▼▼Pork
- Beef
- Rabbit
- ▼Chicken
- ▲Pigeon
- Partridge
- Duck
- Turkey
- ▲▲Fertilized eggs
- ▲▲▲Pheasant

5. Dairy Products
- ▼▼▼Yogurt
- Sour cream
- Sweet cream
- Cream cheese
- Butter
- ▼▼Milk
- Camembert
- ▲Roquefort
- Edam cheese (Dutch)
- ▲▲Goat milk

6. Fruits and Nuts
- ▼▼▼Pineapple
- Papaya
- Mango
- Grapefruit
- Orange
- Banana
- Fig
- Pear
- ▼▼Peach
- Lime
- Melon
- Almond
- Peanut
- Cashew
- Hazel nut
- ▼Olive
- ▲Strawberry
- Chestnut
- Cherry
- ▲▲Apple

7. Miscellaneous	8. Beverages	Water (deep well)
▼▼▼Honey	▼▼▼All sugared	▲Mugwort tea
Molasses	drinks	(yomogi)
▼▼Coconut oil	Tea (containing	Bancha tea
Peanut oil	dye)	(undyed)
Corn oil	Coffee	Chicory tea
Olive oil	Fruit juice	Ohsawa coffee
▼Sunflower oil	Champagne	(yannoh)
Sesame oil	Wine	Grain milk
Canola oil	▼▼Beer	(kokkoh)
Safflower oil	▼Mineral water	▲▲Mu tea
▲Roasted sesame	Carbonated	Dragon tea
oil	water	▲▲Jinseng root tea

---

*All the foods and beverages listed must be natural, never artificially or industrially prepared.

in the greatest quantity—at least 50 to 60 percent of the total amount of food served. Whole grains (unrefined) include: brown rice, wheat, buckwheat, oats, corn, barley, millet, and others. Use them raw, cooked, creamed, with or without water, fried, or baked. Eat as much as you like, provided that you chew thoroughly. Pasta and flours made from whole grains may also be used if naturally grown without chemicals, but these are not the same as what nature provides, the whole grain.

Vegetables

Vegetables and sea vegetables are used to supplement the whole grains but in lesser quantities and less frequently. Use locally grown and seasonal vegetables that are not artificially produced with chemical fertilizers and/or insecticides. Vegetables include carrots, onions, squash, radishes, cabbage, cauliflower, broccoli, lettuce, and a host of others. If you are in any weakened condition, absolutely avoid the most yin vegetables: potatoes, tomatoes, and eggplant.

Sea vegetables such as kombu, wakame, hijiki, nori, and others may be eaten in any area of the country because they agree with our internal environment and because the composition of the ocean is not affected much by the location, season, or weather.

Fish and Other Animal Products

Fish, preferably fresh, is used in even smaller amounts and less often than vegetables but in greater amounts and more often than other animal products.

Fertilized eggs (those that will produce baby chicks) are laid by a hen only after she has been fertilized by a rooster, yet she can and does lay eggs completely on her own. These eggs are non-fertilized eggs, the variety found in most markets and used by the majority of people today. They are lifeless, biologically speaking, and are not recommended. The fertilized egg can be recognized by its small size and its shape—rounded at one end and pointed at the other.

Since macrobiotic practice is not the kind of vegetarianism that is mere sentimentality, hemoglobinic foods are avoided for biological and physiological reasons only. They are avoided in order to develop men who can think.

Animal meat has the ideal composition for an animal; animal glands produce hormones fit for creatures who act only according to their instinct and are unaccustomed to thinking. Anatomically, an animal's center of sensitivity or judgment is not as highly developed as that of man. This is why animals are exploited all their lives by men and finally killed to be eaten.

Those who eat animal products are in a similar manner exploited and often killed by others, for others, or by their own hands. Incidentally, we know of no animal that mobilizes its sons and brothers to kill another nation of creatures as man does. On this point man is insane: his judgment is lower than that of animals.

All men who eat hemoglobinic products depend for sustenance upon animals whose judgment is low and simple. Yet, people who become villains, murderers, liars, or cowards as a result are not to be blamed or punished. They do not realize that their unhappiness is caused by wrong eating and drinking. The fault lies with education, the professional variety, that makes man a phonographic parrot instead of a thinking reed.

In the primary school, ideally speaking, a child should learn to be independent, to think, judge, and act by and for himself. Such training, however, is quite useless if the child does not have a well-developed brain. It is as useless as trying to teach mathematics or reading to a crocodile.

You can control your own behavior by controlling your eating and drinking. You can be your own master or a slave of animal judgment.

In the final analysis, however, there is no need to fear animal products. All depends upon quantity, for quantity changes quality. Anything agreeable becomes disagreeable in excess; the desirable becomes undesirable, even hateful, in immoderate quantities.

Here one can learn the superiority of dialectics as opposed to formal logic. If you know macrobiotic cuisine and its dialectical philosophy, you can yinnize or neutralize food that is too yang (animal products) and avoid the fatal domination of lower judgment (cruel, violent, slavish, delinquent) over higher thinking. You can also yangize or neutralize food that is too yin.

Since you are neither accustomed to pure macrobiotic eating nor in haste to reach satori or infinity, the kingdom of heaven, you may occasionally eat dishes made with animal products provided that the recipes are designed to establish a good balance in your organism by neutralizing too much yang or too much yin. Animal foods are permitted, however, only if they are not contaminated by DDT or chemical additives.

Dairy Products, Fruits, and Nuts

Dairy products, fruits, and nuts are used as pleasure foods and in lesser amounts and less often than animal products. For thousands and thousands of years in China and Japan, and even in India, people lived very happy, peaceful, and long lives without drinking animal milk. Even nowadays, those peoples (more than one billion) drink tea without adding either milk or sugar to it. It might seem to you that they look upon using milk as being sentimentally wrong and are ashamed of being foster brothers and sisters of calves or kids, but this is not true. They avoid milk because they know the biological law prescribed by the principles of the universe, and accept it. Cow's milk is intended to be the nourishment of calves to form their constitution and their fundamental characteristics. There is no reason for man to live upon the milk of the animal, which is biologically and intellectually very inferior to him.

The mortality among children who have been artificially fed animal milk, following the theory of modern nutrition, is plainly higher than among children who have been fostered with human milk. [*Ed.'s note:* Ohsawa wrote this based on his experiences in post-World War II France.] Man may be able to improve the quality of animal milk in the future in order to lower infant mortality, but it will never be possible to turn animal milk into human milk. The biological law cannot be broken. Mortality rates increase as children continue to drink milk and eat dairy products.

The desire among children for animal milk and dairy products is a modern superstition that reveals how much our senses are dulled by taste appeal. This superstition and the exploitation of the senses have a very powerful ally in modern capitalism. The superstition of the senses cannot overshadow biological law, but with advertising and economic power, superstition can violate this law, and very often does. Economic power violates biological and even moral law easily and frequently. The child fed on cow's milk is literally, physiologically, and biologically a little sister or brother of the calf and becomes dull in intellectuality, delicacy, sentimentality, sociability, and spirituality.

Fruits as a category are very yin and can be recommended for the person with a very yang constitution in order to neutralize the injurious residue of a meat diet that has been continued for many long years. In such an instance, they are quite helpful. However, fruits should not be used by sick people with yin constitutions or people in a weakened condition. Those following a basically vegetarian or macrobiotic diet for some time who are not in an overly yang condition do not need much, if any, fruit. Again, if you do eat fruits or nuts, avoid those that are grown at great distances and those that are artificially produced with chemical fertilizers and/or insecticides.

Miscellaneous Foods

Sweeteners, oils, and other miscellaneous foods are used as condiments (or to cook with) and in lesser amounts than other foods. Natural sea salt, soy sauce, and miso are used for cooking and flavor. Also, use only natural spices or chemical seasonings, all commercial Japanese soy sauce and miso included. Yeast is sugar-based and should be eaten in small quantities only or not at all by people with yeast-related illnesses. Baked goods that contain baking soda are not recommended if you are sick or in a weakened condition. The soda promotes rapid rising and expansion in a dough mixture; as such, it is too yin to be part of a balanced, healthful diet for one who is already in an overly yin condition.

Beverages

All drinks, whether yin or yang, are to be used in the smallest quantity of all and the least often. If possible, drink only what your body requires and no more. Bancha tea and natural teas (undyed) are recommended. Do not use tea containing carcinogenic dyes; this includes most varieties that are available commercially. Coffee is prohibited if you are sick or in a weakened condition.

Learning to drink less is much more difficult than learning to eat wisely and simply. But, it is very necessary. Our body weight is about 75 percent water. Cooked rice, for example, contains 60 to 70 percent water; vegetables contain 80 to 90 percent. Thus, we almost invariably take in too much liquid (yin—expansive). To accelerate a macrobiotic cure, you had better drink less . . . enough less so that during a twenty-four-hour period you urinate only two to three times if you are female or three to four times if you are male. It is normal for older folks to urinate two to three additional times per twenty-four hours.

The drink-as-much-as-you-can system is a simple-minded invention because the originator completely ignored the marvelous mechanism of kidney metabolism. He erred in conceiving the kidney to be similar in structure and function to a mechanical sewage system. Large quantities of liquid will flush out and clear a clay or cast iron pipe. The kidney, however, is not a cast iron pipe. It contains tissue that must be flexible and porous so that the processes of filtration, diffusion, and reabsorption can take place.

If liquid is taken in large quantities, the minute openings in the semi-permeable kidney tissue decrease in size (these openings are surrounded by tissue that is spongelike, that soaks up liquid and swells) and little or no liquid can pass through. For all practical purposes, the kidneys are blocked. The net result is a complete reversal of what the drink-as-much-as-you-can system intended.

Help your tired, overworked kidneys. Drink less.

WAYS OF EATING AND DRINKING

Chewing

Chew every mouthful of food at least fifty times. If you wish to assimilate the macrobiotic philosophy as quickly as possible, chew each mouthful one hundred to one hundred and fifty times. The most tasty morsel becomes more so if chewed well. The foods that are good and necessary for your body become so delectable that you will not give them up until the end of your days. Try chewing a piece of steak carefully. You will very rapidly find it to be tasteless.

Art of Macrobiotic Cooking

Our macrobiotic cuisine, which can be so very delicious, requires a creative cook who also understands the art of yin-yang balance. Unfortunately, modern education neglects the creative capacity to such a degree that it is rare that we meet a good cook. Yet, to live is to create. Without creation, we cannot exist, for our bodies create blood from our daily intake of food and beverages. Blood creates or motivates all our activities. Human adaptability is itself a result of this creative capacity.

Life is the expression of creativity and, in turn, depends completely on the composition, proportion, preparation, and order of yin and yang elements in our eating and drinking.

Being a stranger to macrobiotic cooking, you will prepare

From Sickly Boy
to Wrestler

One summer, my dad took us all to upstate New York to a macro-biotic summer camp. I was only ten at the time, and I can remember somebody talking about George Ohsawa. He can do great things; he's been everywhere; etc. It didn't mean too much to me. People used to say George was up at six o'clock in the morning on his hands and knees, scrubbing the kitchen floors. I figured this guy's a kook or something.

Anyway, my mom and dad wanted to get us kids up there so that George could analyze us and say what we should eat or shouldn't eat. I was pretty sickly at the time. He looked at us and said, "Being so young, you can become better if you eat the right foods." My mom and dad had the list.

Using Ohsawa's way of eating, I became a successful colle-giate wrestler. Whole grains and fresh vegetables still give me all the energy I need.

Michael Smith
Son of Dick and Penny Smith

foods that are not so delicious at first. Never mind. Under these circumstances you will eat less—a vacation for your tired stomach and intestines. My congratulations.

Furthermore, your beginning meals will probably not be very well balanced. There is no need to worry, however. Through practice and the study of macrobiotic theory, your judgment will develop rapidly; you will soon be a master of the art of balancing yin and yang elements in food preparation—the most basic art in your life.

Yin and yang vary according to the climate of origin and the season of the year. Further, the yin and yang characteristics of food can be greatly influenced by preparation and manner of eating. This is why cooking and table manners are so important. (In old Japan, eating and drinking were considered to be ceremonies of paramount importance—the creation of life and thinking.)

Bear in mind that the invention of fire, without which we could not cook, has a very deep meaning: It marks the point at which the path of man diverged from that of all other animals.

Transmutation

The great effectiveness of the macrobiotic method is rooted in the process of transmutation, without which nature as we know it (the human organism included) could not exist. Simply stated, transmutation occurs when one element is changed into another, either naturally or artificially. This process, known and understood thousands of years ago by the sages of the world, enabled them to produce gold from other elements and to achieve combinations of metals and other substances that modern science can only duplicate with great difficulty, progress and mechanical devices notwithstanding.

I have always taught my students that they can transmute themselves from arrogant, diseased, materialistic men into humble, healthy, spiritual beings; that instead of being happy in appearance only and being killed by accident, murder, or microbes or at the very least ending their lives as professional slaves, they can enjoy infinite freedom, eternal happiness, and absolute justice for many long years. Now, after many years of effort on my part, there is proof that biochemical transmutation is neither the mystique of the alchemists of old nor just an abstract philosophical concept. It is a practical, living, verifiable reality.

On June 21, 1964, in Tokyo, I completed the transmutation of the element sodium (Na) into potassium (K) under laboratory conditions of low temperature, pressure, and energy. This significant achievement comes as a bombshell to science, for until now, this type of reaction was thought possible only under conditions available in a high-energy particle accelerator. Our results were obtained, however, through the use of only a twenty-centimeter vacuum tube and a mere one hundred watts of power! (Further scientific evidence that substantiates the theory of biochemical transmutation is to be found in the revolutionary works of M. Louis Kervran, a French research biologist. Our chance meeting in 1960 led directly to the startling event of June 21.)

The great significance of this discovery is twofold:

1. It indicates that biochemical transmutation of elements is possible using the minute amounts of energy available in the human organism.

2. It is a verification of the foundation stone of macrobiotic philosophy, namely the understanding that through the process of transmutation, our bodies can produce all that they need for health from the simple diet that is a result of an understanding of the structure of the universe and its order.

Now, at last, what we have instinctively and intuitively known for thousands of years can be demonstrated in the laboratory. In order to maintain natural health, man must not borrow elements from nature as he does when he doses himself with specifics such as iron, calcium, vitamin C, and sugar substitutes, to name only a few. He must be independent and manufacture his needs within his organism, by and for himself.

A cow, for example, eats only grasses, yet it has a very strong bone structure. Where does the calciumthat is required for these healthy bones come from? Certainly not directly from the grass, a particularly poor source of that element. It is, however, a rich source of potassium. Hydrogen is present in the cow's drinking water. The formula below outlines the natural, internal production of calcium in an organism through biological transmutation:

$$K^{39} + H^1 + \text{internal heat (activity)} \text{ - forms - } Ca^{40}$$

There is no reason to believe that the process in a human being would not be similar.

Human beings have digestive organs that can transmute chlorophyll into hemoglobin. In fact, all of what we eat is either transformed into blood (the prime source of raw material for our instant-by-instant re-creation of ourselves) or it is eliminated. For us, laboratory-produced calcium (inorganic because it is not the result of a living process) contaminates the blood and can be fatal.

In the process of biochemical transmutation, the most essential ingredient is activity, the by-products of which are oxygen and heat. (Activity keeps both the boa constrictor and the lizard alive under the high temperatures that are found in their natural habitats. If we immobilize either of these creatures experimentally, it rapidly dies.) The natural tendency on the part of an average child to be tremendously active is very favorable to the maintenance of good health provided that his diet is simple and well-balanced in its yin and yang elements.

Where there is too much salt and little activity, there is no growth. With activity (a necessary element in transmutation) at a minimum, the conversion of raw materials from a balanced diet into what the body requires is upset. Elements other than calcium are produced, deficiencies result, and growth is arrested.

The process of transmutation goes on wherever there is life, no matter what sort of diet we follow. By understanding how it works, we can truly be the creators of ourselves and our existence. This is why my philosophy is called the philosophy of transmutation. Everything changes—illness becomes health, health becomes illness—and so on into infinity.

Maintaining Balance

It is further advisable to choose foods from Table 1 that are at or reasonably near the mid-point between extreme yin and extreme yang within each category, unless there is a specific reason for another choice. This is the delicate balance point at which the greatest health and happiness can be achieved.

I cannot over-emphasize the point that macrobiotic living is not rigid adherence to a set of rules. The maintenance of a healthy balance in our daily lives demands from each individual an adaptability and an awareness of the constantly changing influences of

An Everyday Guy

I met George for the second time at a summer camp in California when I was twelve, This time, I saw him personally. He was there for a couple of days with Lima. My brother, the de Langre kids, and I were out picking raspberries off the bushes and we came back with our shirts stuffed full of raspberries. Somebody said, "Go ask Ohsawa if he wants some." He figured Ohsawa was really going to yell at us and tell us we were wrong for eating all those raspberries.

So I said, "Okay," and I walked up to old George and said, "Do you want some raspberries?"

And he laughed and smiled and with a big grin on his face said, "Ah so, very good, very good. Eat many!" He took a handful and started eating them.

I know he was an idol to many people, but I knew him as just a normal everyday guy.

Michael Smith
Son of Dick and Penny Smith

many factors. This makes a happy and healthy existence a full-time job.

The type of climate one lives in and the sort of activity one is engaged in determine what and how one eats. (Factors such as place of birth, the type of constitution one has, the season of the year, as well as many other things are taken into consideration as one's comprehension of the Order of the Universe grows.) For instance, the man who lives in a cold climate needs foods that are slightly more yang than those necessary for one who inhabits the tropics, while the person who works in the fields can tolerate slightly more yin food than can he whose work confines him to a desk. Everything is relative to and is determined by each individual person, for no set of rules can possibly cover all the variations that exist from one person to the next.

The phrase "more yang" should not be construed to mean a diet based wholly on meat, just as "more yin" does not imply meals that are made up of mostly fruits and sugar. The fact that one's daily intake of food is based preponderantly on whole grains, however, is taken for granted.

With the improvement in your health and happiness that results from your growing comprehension of yin-yang theory, expand your food choices slowly and carefully if you are curious or adventurous. From time to time, you can measure your health and happiness by means of the self-consultation that utilizes the Seven Conditions of Health starting on page 35.

Everyone is born happy. If an individual does not continue to be happy, it is his own fault; through ignorance, he has violated the Order of the Universe through improper eating and drinking.

If you wish to live a happy, interesting, amusing, joyful, and long life, you should strengthen your comprehension and unveil your supreme judging ability by eating simple and natural food.

THE MAGNIFICENCE OF OLD AGE

At the age of forty, I was startled to feel weakness in my body. "I am beginning to get old," I thought, since in Japan it is said that old age begins when pain and stiffness appear, somewhere between the ages of forty and forty-five.

My feeling of age was not the result of macrobiotic living but because of the circumstances of my early life. As a youth, I had lived and eaten poorly, studying all the time. Later, I worked as a sailor on the Indian Ocean. My Arabian crewmates, raised in a tropical country and possessing very strong constitutions, thrived on the hard work we did. I had grown up in a much different climate so the combination of ocean, labor, and diet not only made me very sickly but caused what I felt to be "old age."

After my very long voyage, I returned to Japan and recovered my strength by eating delicious brown rice. From that time on, I have never felt tired, nor have I ever had the need to rest. In fact, as long as I am awake, I am at work. I easily fulfill three of the conditions for good health:

1. No fatigue
2. Good appetite
3. Good sleep

How could I feel anything but gratitude for my years of macrobiotic living?

The first ten years were full of mistakes. Sometimes, I took too much salt; at other times, not enough. I experienced much failure. Though the last five years of my long stay in Paris were spent under the poorest of living conditions, I have now re-established good health. I can now enjoy any cuisine—Western, Chinese, Japanese, or Indian. I like fruit, candy, chocolate, and whiskey very much. If I choose these things now, I am able to avoid harm by balancing their yin and yang qualities.

I have told you this because many people think that macrobiotic practice is a twentieth century variety of stoicism. But he who cannot eat and drink whatever he chooses is a cripple. Macrobiotic living is a way to build health that enables us to eat and drink anything we like, whenever we like, without being obsessed or driven to do so. Macrobiotic practice is not a negative way of living. It is positive, creative, artistic, religious, and philosophical.

Macrobiotically speaking, old age begins at seventy. At this time an individual should:

1. Reduce salt intake.
2. Make certain that his daily food is as simple and natural as possible.
3. Use vegetable oils daily in small amounts.

The macrobiotic guideline for old age amounts to simply this: "live in nature." Enjoy cold in winter, accept heat in summer, admire flowers in spring, and write poems in autumn. Live in nature with a calm, quiet spirit. Give to others of your happiness, for old age is the most happy time of life.

I recall a very fitting poem by the German poet Lautenbach. It describes an oak tree that has withstood several hundred years of buffeting by all kinds of weather—wind, rain, storm, frost, and snow. It is a very tall tree with wide, strong branches and many leaves that sparkle in the sunshine and flutter in every breeze. It gives much shade and provides a fine resting place for travelers. It is an image of God, a joyful achievement. It is the product of a life of hammering by nature's hardships. Its quiet magnificence whispers the secret of life. The privilege of having an old age such as this is given to those who practice macrobiotic living.

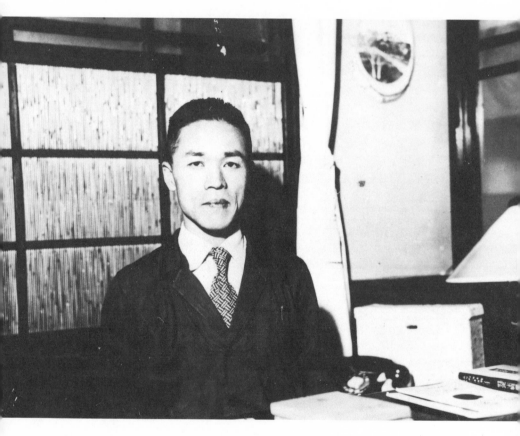

George Ohsawa at his desk at the Kumasawa Trading Company in Japan, 1918.

2

HEALTH
AND DISEASE

SEVEN CONDITIONS OF HEALTH

Before observing my dietetic directions, it would be wise for you
to evaluate the state of your health in accordance with the seven
conditions that follow.

The first three conditions are physiological; if you satisfy them
all, you score fifteen points or five points for each. The fourth, fifth,
and sixth, psychological in nature, are valued at ten points each.
The seventh and most important condition of all is worth fifty-five
points. In all, there are a total of one hundred points.

Those who score more than forty points at first are in relatively
good health. Should you total sixty points in three months, it will
be a great success for you.

Be sure to do this self-consultation before you try a macrobiotic
diet and again at the beginning of each month following. In this
way, you will be able to check your progress and the rigor of your
application.

Try this test on your friends. You will be surprised to find that
some of them are actually in very poor health although their
outward appearance may be quite good.

1. No Fatigue: You should not feel fatigued. If you catch cold,

your organism has been tired for many years. Even one cold in ten years is a bad sign for there is no bird or insect that ever catches cold, even in cold countries and cold weather. The root of your disease is therefore very deep.

If you are prone to saying, "It is too difficult," "It is impossible," or "I am not prepared for such a thing," you reveal the extent of your problem. If you are really healthy, you can overpower and chase away difficulties one after the other as a dog chases a rabbit. If you ever try to avoid difficulties, however, you are a defeatist.

We must be adventurers in life since today unceasingly advances into tomorrow, the unknown. The bigger the difficulty, the bigger the pleasure. This attitude is the sign of freedom from fatigue.

Fatigue is the real foundation of all diseases. You can cure it without any medicine if you understand and practice the macrobiotic way to longevity and rejuvenation.

2. Good Appetite: If you cannot take the simplest food with joy, pleasure, and deep gratitude to God the Creator, your appetite is poor. If you find simple brown bread or cooked whole brown rice very appetizing, you have a good appetite and a healthy, strong stomach. A good appetite for food and sex is health itself.

   Sexual appetite and joyful satisfaction are essential conditions of happiness. If a man or woman has no appetite for sex and experiences no pleasure, he or she is estranged from the dialectical law of life, yin and yang. Violation of this law through ignorance can only lead to sickness and depression.

3. Deep and Good Sleep: If you dream or speak in your sleep, your rest is not deep and good. If your sleep is healthy, four to six hours of it satisfies you entirely. If you cannot fall asleep within three or four minutes after putting your head on the pillow, under any circumstance, at any time, your mind is not free from some fear. Your sleep has been imperfect if you cannot awaken spontaneously at an hour predetermined by you before retiring.

Physical Flexibility

George Ohsawa impressed me in many ways. One of them was his physical flexibility. He used to like to show off his ability to bend his neck right and left far enough to rest his ears on his shoulders. He could also turn his head left and right in order to look behind him without turning his body. This degree of flexibility is fairly unknown in the western world except among birds.

Another of his characteristics that made a memorable impression on me was the quality of his voice. It was very low, a baritone, and clear. His body was so clean that, even though he spoke in a low tone, his voice reverberated through his body as though through a sound board, carrying to a great distance. I remember one day in Martha's Vineyard when Ohsawa was talking to a small group of friends in the living room. I had an errand to do outside at some distance from the house. Even though I was far away, I could still hear his voice and discern his words distinctly. It was quite amazing to me.

Cecile Levin
Macrobiotic teacher and counselor

4. Good Memory: Memory is the single most important factor in our lives, the foundation of our personality, the compass of our being. Without a strong memory, without a storehouse of varied memories, we are nothing but machines. For example, very young children, fascinated by fire and unable to resist the impulse to touch it, eventually get burned. The memory of this experience usually causes them to handle fire with care for the rest of their lives. Therefore, human behavior, if it is not to end in misfortune, depends on sound judgment. Sound judgment, in turn, depends on remembered experience.

Since the capacity to remember increases with age, it is possible to improve our memory infinitely, even to the extent

of not forgetting anything that we see or hear. We can thus
avoid the miserable feeling that comes from not remembering
those who have been kind to us.

Through my macrobiotic directions, you can re-establish
and infinitely strengthen this faculty.

5. Good Humor: A man of good health is free from anger, fear,
    or suffering and is cheerful and pleasant under all circum-
    stances. The more difficulties and enemies he has, the more
    happy, brave, and enthusiastic he becomes.

    Your appearance, voice, behavior, and even your criti-
    cism should distribute deep gratitude and thankfulness to all
    those who are in your presence. All your words should be
    expressive of a deep gratitude, like the singing of birds and
    insects or the poems of Tagore. The stars, the sun, the moun-
    tains, rivers, and seas are all ours. How can we exist without
    being happy? We should be full of delight like a boy who has
    just received a magnificent present. If we are not, we lack
    good health and are particularly deficient in this fifth condi-
    tion, good humor. The healthy person never gets angry.

    How many intimate friends have you? A large number
    and variety of them indicate a profoundly deep comprehen-
    sion of the universe. Parents, brothers, and sisters are not
    friends, as such. A friend is he whom you like, admire, and
    respect; he who likes and admires you; he who helps you to
    realize your fondest dreams at all costs, forever, without
    being asked.

    How many dear friends have you? If the number is few,
    you are a very exclusive person or a sad delinquent without
    enough good humor to make others happy. If, however, you
    have more than two billion intimate friends, you can say that
    you are a friend of all mankind. It is not sufficient if your
    intimate friends include only human beings, living or dead.
    You will have to love and admire all beings and things,
    including grains of sand, drops of water, and blades of grass.

    If you cannot make your wife or children into intimate
    friends, you are very sick. If you are not cheerful under any
    circumstances, you are a blind man who sees neither this

limited world of relativity nor the infinite, absolute universe, both full of marvels. If you have any complaint, be it mental, moral, physiological, or social, shut yourself in a private room like the shellfish and speak out your sorrow to yourself alone.

6. Clarity in Thinking and Doing: Those people in good health should have the ability to think, judge, and act with promptness and clarity. Promptness is the expression of freedom. Those who are prompt, quick, precise, and ready to answer any challenge or necessity are healthy.

   They distinguish themselves by their ability to establish order everywhere. This orderliness can be observed throughout the animal and vegetable kingdoms. Beauty of action or form is an expression of the comprehension of the Order of the Universe. Health and happiness, wholesomeness and holiness are also expressions of the order translated into our daily lives. Divinity, eternity, health, and life are one.

7. The Mood of Justice: Those persons with a complete understanding of justice have reached satori, for justice = health = supreme judgment = oneness = infinity = satori. They know the traditional philosophy of the Far East in all its profundity and have earned a full one hundred points in our self-evaluation test.

   If, however, you have not reached this level, you can still earn fifty-five points, provided that justice is not merely a concept or idea about which you only dream. If you are actively involved in coming to know what it represents, if every day brings you closer to a full understanding of the order of nature, if your intention or goal is to grasp the deepest meaning of the traditional philosophy of the Far East, you have caught the mood of justice. Your growing comprehension will lead to self-realization and merits fifty-five points.

   The mood of justice is revealed by your tendency to live in accordance with the natural Order of the Universe, by your inclination to recognize yin and yang in every phenomenon, be it physical, mental, or spiritual, on every level of daily life such as eating, drinking, thinking, judging, doing, speaking, buying, selling, reading, walking, and working.

In other words, you should live the biological law: From one grain, ten thousand grains. All vegetables and animals return ten thousand times more than they receive. One grain is given to the earth; the earth gives back ten thousand grains. One silkworm fed by man gives hundreds of thousands of eggs plus ten thousand yards of silk yarn. Some female fish give billions of eggs. Such is the natural biological law.

If your parents have given you life and have fed you to the age of ten, take care of them infinitely, ten times ten thousand. When they are gone, help the parents of others directly through your own action or indirectly through other means. This is the Far Eastern concept of "On" that has been completely misunderstood in the West. It is not merely the repayment of a debt. It is far more than that. "On" is joyfulness in distributing infinite freedom and eternal happiness; it is justice or the absolute joy of life.

Justice, at first glance, would appear to have no connection whatever with diet. It might seem that diet, a practicality, has been replaced by a useless abstraction similar to those that have plagued other philosophies for thousands of years. This is misleading, for diet is justice and justice is diet; they are one. To follow the macrobiotic way is to come to know justice; by the same token, to know justice is to follow the macrobiotic way, the order of nature or life itself.

Since nature has provided us with foods that are proper for our bodies, we can achieve health by recognizing and using them. This is macrobiotic living, the materialization of the order of nature in our eating and drinking. If we live according to this order, health can result; if we are ignorant of it, unhappiness and disease are more likely to follow. This is simple, clear, and practical. It is true justice.

The seven conditions outlined above cannot be realized without strictly observing my simple macrobiotic directions. Through them, you can be the creator of your own life, health, and happiness without relying on others; you can be independent and free.

THE SEVEN STAGES OF DISEASE

According to Far Eastern medicine, we may consider the stages of disease as follows:

1. Fatigue: caused by a disorderly life (undisciplined, mean, ungrateful) or a chaotic family or parents.
2. Pain and suffering: caused by low judgment (capricious, sensorial, sentimental, conceptual, exclusive) and psychosomatic illness.
3. Chronic symptoms: caused by an excess of yin or yang in food (through love or hate of certain foods), leading to headache, painful chest, diarrhea, vomiting, ulcer, trachoma, leukemia (all skin and blood diseases).
4. Sympatheticotonic or vagotonic: The sickness has ascended to the autonomic nervous system.
5. Functional and structural changes in the organs themselves.
6. Psychological or emotional: schizophrenia, neurasthenia, hysteria, cardiac dilation, etc.
7. Spiritual disease: This afflicts those of such good physical constitution that they bypass the first six stages. They suffer unconsciously from their arrogance and intolerance, and despite the appearance of success are without faith, hope, joy, or love, and their lives always end tragically.

All of these diseases are often interconnected. They are difficult to classify, but every disease may be approximately localized in one or another of the stages we are now going to discuss. Their classification is according to the tree of diseases: The root (stage 1) is a disordered, weak, and ungrateful life; the trunk (stage 2) represents low judging ability; the branches are stages 3 and 4; the flowers of the disease are stage 5; the fruits of the disease are stages 6 and 7.

Stage 1 prepares the physiological illness for at least ten years.

Stage 2 represents the disease's germination (cold, weariness). Stage 3 appears more or less abruptly, but has already been in preparation for many years (thrombosis, sunstroke). Stage 4 is the end of vagotonia or sympatheticotonia. It is during stage 5 that grievous illnesses of body structures or organs (teeth, eyes, heart) and their deformation or destruction develop. Stage 6 includes paranoia, emotivity, easy loss of temper, restlessness, silence, lack of sociability, total lack of patience, exclusiveness, etc.

It is obvious that elementary diseases such as those in stages 1, 2, and 3 are much easier to heal than those in the higher stages. The chief difficulty lies in an intolerant mind.

In any disease, one must begin with the most elementary stage: an unruly, cowardly, and ungrateful life. That is to say that one must first of all learn the principle of *vivere parvo*, eating and drinking only what is absolutely necessary in order to produce an independent and autonomous life. Without treating the disease from its root, one will achieve no fundamental healing.

Our physiological progression must develop in a direction that is quite opposed to that of disease. But many people develop in the same direction as illness, misguided by modern professional materialistic education and medication. Nowadays, many students drop out of their studies after suffering tuberculosis, nervousness, etc. This is unfortunately a form of natural selection. This is the struggle for life. But rather than merely protecting ill students, there is a need to do away with the kind of education that produces such students. In this way, much can be saved.

I like and wonder at the English spirit of sportmanship and the frontier spirit of the Americans. But at the present time, the really strong one must be and can be the happy victor—absolute justice being the strongest. The really strong one can be produced only by supreme judging ability. Ancient Far Eastern medicine is the very technique to produce biologically and physiologically strong people, provided with a solid logic, following the Unifying Principle. But this principle was lost long ago. Modern medicine is partly responsible for this because it has forgotten or ignored the Unifying Principle theory. Theory without practice is of no worth; practice without theory is dangerous. The old Far Eastern medicine has been wiped out by the young modern medicine, which has a great many symptomatic instruments. Whatever has a beginning has an end. Far Eastern physicians who knew the Unifying Principle have disappeared, and diseases proliferate.

THE MYSTERY OF HEALTH

There are a great many mysteries. For instance, little birds are covered with feathers. They can fly easily in any direction (much better than a plane whose roaring is so unpleasant) and always sing in so charming a way. What wonderful beings.

A tiny grain absorbs a little water, opens, pushes up small leaves, and grows day after day into a mature plant, which in its turn gives grains by the thousands. This is also a mystery. Why does this tiny grain absorb water? By what process? This is still an enigma.

But look at the sun, that grand and flaming ball. Why does it not fall? Why does it expend so much energy? Why has it for centuries swung up there above our heads? Nobody is able to fully answer these questions. All these things are mysteries. Not a single mystery has been revealed since the beginning of our world. What we have learned for thousands of years is just a geometrical point, infinitely tiny in the presence of all these mysteries.

But there is still another mystery, nearer at hand, that affects us all, namely: man, the greatest mystery. He himself contains multitudes of mysteries. Should you be able to understand him, everything would become understandable. Why and how is his heat produced continuously, night and day? Who or what controls it? What is the process of cardiac automatism? What is the chemical process that works constantly through the whole of life to transform proteins in the stomach? How does man's memory work?

An even greater mystery is the question of what precedes memory. It is the very foundation of our knowledge. Our comprehension, our judgment, our expression, our thinking, our actions, all depend on it. It is called *tabula rasa*. This is another name for mystery itself.

Curing My Back Pain

After his lecture, I was so shy I couldn't go up to George—I was afraid to face him. So I waited until everyone had left and finally only he and I were standing there. When he became aware of me, he said, "How can I help you?"

And I said, "I have had lower back trouble for over ten years. Orthopedics have wanted to remove discs. I even went to a specialist who injected a sodium solution into my ligaments to try to strengthen them."

He just shook his head and said, "That can't help you; injecting a liquid (yin) is not the answer to cure an overly yin condition."

So I asked him if I could cure it by macrobiotic methods and he said, "Very easily. You must eat nothing but brown rice for two months. I'll guarantee you that you'll be completely cured."

And then he saw my sanpaku eyes, a very yin condition indicated by white showing on three sides of the eyeball. And then he came closer to me and saw that my nose was very purple. He said, "Very, very yin."

And I said, "Mr. Ohsawa, I have been eating nothing but fruits and vegetables for the past few months."

And he said, "Your condition is very dangerous." So I thanked him, went back to my little hotel room, and gave away all the food I had. That's when I started macrobiotics.

Alex Lesnevsky
Retired from Chico-San, Inc.

Life is full of mysteries.

Modern physiology is on the track of another mystery: the vegetative nervous system, which is composed of two antagonistic systems, sympathetic and parasympathetic. The sympathetic nerve can expand, and it busies itself with every dilation and expansion of all tissues and organs in our body. On the contrary, the parasympathetic nerve controls every constriction. This one carries a yang, centripetal energy, whereas the other has yin, centrifugal energy. Our body is, then, under the influence of two antagonistic fundamental forces: yin and yang. They are the two hands which give life to all our organs. Now we are on the track of this unknown: man.

Health is nothing but a good equilibrium established between these two antagonistic systems. Illness is, then, nothing but a transient or chronic imbalance between these two opposing forces. Transitory imbalance is expressed by diseases of stages 1 or 2, whereas the chronic variety is indicated by all other stages of illness.

One must establish a good equilibrium between the two systems to enjoy good health. But what is the reason for imbalance? Of course, it comes fundamentally from our diet. An excess of yin foods makes the sympathetic system predominate, whereas too yang a diet gives pre-eminence to the parasympathetic system. But at the very first, it is yin that animates yang and, in the long run, or in excess, yin neutralizes yang and fortifies yin and vice versa.

We are just puppets, animated by these two nervous systems. In this respect, we are not at all autonomous unless we learn to control this balance by our daily diet. Then, we can be our own masters.

What my preparatory dietetic instructions recommend is to establish a good balance between these two antagonistic systems. Being a summation of my long studies, my preparatory directions are suitable for all and can, with specific ailments, establish good health in a general way after a period of practice.

After all, our health, our happiness, our liberty, and our comprehension depend physiologically upon a good balance between the two nervous systems. At the same time, equilibrium depends mentally on the concept of the Order of the Universe, which we will study in Part Two.

3

COMPLETELY NATURAL CURING

THE SECRET MEDICINE

Severe tuberculosis eliminated in two months by Mr. Wago; a thirty-year-old case of leprosy overcome by Mr. Tsutsumi; colitis cured by General Matsui in three weeks; a combination of asthma and skin disease that had lasted for forty years gone in one month; cancer of the womb, cancer of the breast, rheumatism, arthritis, poliomyelitis, female baldness and infertility, the inability to speak, tuberculosis of the spine and kidney . . . I have been witnessing the disappearance of these and many other diseases for many years in those individuals who have deeply understood macrobiotic living.

The thought of all the people who have been saved by macrobiotic living in the past, plus the fact that I too was rescued from certain death many years ago, makes me feel nothing less than endless gratitude and thankfulness every day.

A very few people, possibly one in ten, do not respond in the usual one to two months. They have come to macrobiotic living too late and unfortunately cannot be helped. They have waited much too long before seeking help and are regrettably destined to die.

It is usually so easy to help the sick that I am amazed when I think about it. I then wonder why so many people (including my-

Master of Macrobiotic

*In 1945, after the Japanese military government had declared complete
surrender, Ohsawa was released from jail. He had been jailed during
World War II for his anti-war writings. I attended his first seminar
held after the war and my heart was deeply saddened to see Ohsawa
almost blind due to his living conditions in jail. When I saw him, he
was wearing sunglasses and using a stick to help himself walk. However, his spirit was as high as ever.*

*During the lecture he said, "The best healing method is following
the most basic diet: eating brown rice, miso soup, and radish pickles
only. One can heal all sicknesses with this simple diet." This he knew
because of his own experience. He called one who followed such a diet,
"a master of macrobiotic."*

Noboru Sakaguchi
Owner of TAMA,
a European macrobiotic distributor

self) fall ill in the first place and why they tolerate suffering for so
long.

The answer is a simple one: We are all ignorant of the simple,
clear relationship between food and life. Anyone who understands
this basic macrobiotic teaching knows how foolish it is to become
ill; with such knowledge, one can be sick no more. Yet at times I
think that it would be interesting to be sick once again because it
has been many years since I suffered last.

In macrobiotic healing, we never use medicine; our pharmacy
is the kitchen. My method is based on the potency of daily food-
simple things like brown rice, carrots, onions, radishes, burdock
root, miso, and sea vegetables.

How such commonplace foods can affect so many strange
ailments and eliminate them in one or two months is very puzzling

to people with a scientific orientation. "Why do so many desperately weakened victims thrive on it?" they ask. "What is the secret?"

When a man falls ill, his friends offer the usual sympathetic advice. "Take it easy, eat some good food, rest . . ."

But illness is not a precious jewel. If we nurture it, we preserve it for a long time. The disease—not the human being—must be thrown away like the useless thing that it is.

In theory, we all know that we live because we eat. Not one of us, however, seems to have a practical answer to the important questions:

- What is the right food?
- What is the right quantity?
- What is the right method of preparation?
- What is the right manner in which to eat?

Given the right food, we can live a happy, healthy, peaceful life. Given food that is not right, we are no longer right men—we are inhuman beings. We become weak, sick, poor, incapable of working—joyless.

What then is the right food?

If our approach is analytical, this is a very difficult question to answer. Protein, fats, carbohydrates, vitamins, minerals, calories—so many things to consider. No one as yet has given a concrete, livable answer to our question in this way, not even scientists, scholars, or specialists.

Take protein, for instance. Are there two experts who agree about the kind and quality needed by human beings?

Vitamins and minerals are in the same category. People say, "Apples are good for you." But who tells us how many ounces to eat, when to eat them, and how to prepare an apple properly so that it is fit for us to consume? Are apples good for every person, all the time?

I know of one boy who ate too many apples and eventually died of children's dysentery. An elementary school teacher died after eating thirty-two apples in four days on the advice of her physician. One famous doctor of nutrition, a great believer in the effectiveness of apples, died recently from an excess of them. I could go on and on—the list of casualties from food abuse is a very long one.

There obviously is a right amount for everything. "Too much of even a good thing is not wise." But who knows what is too much?

Vitamin C is supposedly very important for good nutrition. How much and how often? Since no two people have the same constitution or character, since everyone's physical condition is different, can we establish a standard amount that would be practical in every situation? We suspect that whoever seeks this answer is running a fool's errand.

But what if by some strange miracle the experts were able to determine the right amount? Some nations might not be capable of producing enough of it to supply an entire population. Some places could not store enough for everyone. And many individuals could not afford the price of their basic needs.

It is so difficult to apply such a theory practically and even theoretically. There must be a simpler way.

Throughout history, men have lived happy lives without complicated analytical concepts of nutrition. Although our ancestors gave little thought to apples, they were healthier, happier, and wiser than we are. Even beasts seem to be able to live joyfully without concerning themselves with chemistry or scientific detail. Perhaps, there is hope for us too.

We are so far removed from simplicity. We hear and read things like this: "Lack of scientific information and illness go hand-in-hand." "Health is the result of research; research costs money; money is therefore essential to health."

But what about the millions of people in the history of the world who led full lives long before science became so important, and on much less money than we spend today?

"Animal protein and calcium are basic to good nutrition." Isn't it curious that a cow can produce not only the meat and milk that we feel is so essential for us but her own massive bone structure as well from a diet of grasses alone?

If the modern, superstitious belief in science, money, and meat is a valid one, how miserable we are. A poor man is forever excluded—he can neither be healthy nor enjoy his life. Existence is no more than a game of chance in which the cards are stacked in favor of the rich, the educated, the knowledgeable.

It cannot be that God would create anything so unfair. Anybody can live joyfully in health.

If we compare the food that we eat today with that of our ancestors, we are struck by the vast difference between the two. So important a staple as whole rice was once cultivated with natural fertilizers while today the laboratory supplies them. We begin to suspect that the biggest problem lies in the area of what is natural and what is unnatural.

Few of us question the fact that it is natural for man to be born, to be active, to grow. And we agree that it is natural to depend upon food for life and survival. At this point, however, we fail to see the obvious.

Of all things that grow on a farm, the strongest seem to be the natural grasses—the weeds. The farmer easily spends as much time and effort eliminating them as he does cultivating his produce—and still they grow again and again naturally, by themselves, in the face of every chemical obstacle. Any farmer who has battled weeds will agree that they are more resistant than anything he grows for human consumption.

Here is the clue to successful existence. The ingenuity of science is juvenile as compared to the quietly irresistible force with which nature animates the entire universe.

- To live and be active, man depends upon food;
- To live naturally, he must eat natural food;
- If he lives naturally, a man can be healthy and happy.

Since man is a natural product of a natural environment, he must live as close to nature as possible; to be healthy and happy he must eat natural foods. But what are natural foods? They are the ones that our ancestors have used for a thousand years. And they differ from one country and climate to the next. This is why there are so many nationalities, religions, societies, and customs.

One might say that macrobiotic teaching is rooted in the concept of principal food. It is a reaffirmation and reapplication of the ancient wisdom and has produced the miraculous results that lead to an inevitable conclusion: we must re-evaluate, relearn, and apply the concept of principal food in our daily lives. We must know that natural food is important and know the reasons why it is vital to our present and future well-being. Otherwise, we are unqualified to be healthy, happy, and peaceful.

This is the secret of macrobiotic healing.

MY NATURAL MEDICINE

What Is My Therapy?

According to Far Eastern macrobiotic medicine, there is no need for therapeutics or remedies because the mother of all life in the universe, Nature herself, is the greatest healer. All disease, unhappiness, crime, and punishment result from behavior that violates the Order of the Universe.

The cure is, therefore, infinitely simple. Merely stop violating that order and allow Nature to do her miraculous work.

All disease can be cured completely in ten days, according to my philosophical conception of the world and of the structure of the universe. All disease is located in or fed by our blood. Since we decompose one-tenth of that blood every day at a rate of three hundred thousand globules per second, it should be entirely transformed and completely renewed in a matter of months if we follow a natural way of eating and drinking. What is natural is determined by the consideration of both the innate biological needs of the human organism and the needs that are superimposed by type of activity and environmental conditions such as weather, altitude, and time of year.

Although the theory and its logic are quite understandable, the technique of its application is delicate and can be very complex. In keeping with the traditional Far Eastern belief that no theory without a practical technique is useful and that no technique without an uncomplicated, clear theory is safe, my therapy is very simple:

1. Natural food
2. No medicine
3. No surgery
4. No inactivity

Again, theory is simple in my ages-old philosophy yet its application in our daily lives can be as complicated as our modern kitchens, agriculture, and industry have become. Everything depends upon your understanding and accuracy.

Diet and Health

Our civilization, one of abundance and abuse, approves of eating large amounts of food. A particular theory of nutrition which dates back hardly a hundred years recommends that we eat not only thousands of calories but also consume a certain percentage of animal protein each day. Yet in Asia hundreds of millions of "non-civilized" people have lived successfully as vegetarians for thousands of years.

Man is free. He can eat defeated, weak, innocent, defenseless beings. Perhaps the latter were born to feed the strong, as the militants of "survival of the fittest" affirm. Well, to each his own— a man's menu can be as varied as his whims.

But I would like to give you some advice. It is the conclusion I have reached after fifty years of studying and teaching the Order of the Universe. In my opinion, it is the key to the awareness of the fact that we are always in the kingdom of heaven. It can enable you to immunize yourself your entire life against any disease—cancer and mental illness included. The secret is quite simple: avoid animal protein as much as possible, and completely avoid refined sugar. Refined sugar and excess animal protein are the two main causes of all of our misfortunes.

You may enjoy animal protein in small quantities. But do not forget that, in accordance with the teachings of the ancient sages, billions of Asians lived well and avoided animal protein for many thousands of years in China and India. One can live without meat and fish. Neither is necessary. But I repeat, you may eat them for the sake of pleasure. However, restrict your intake if you wish to preserve your physical and mental health. Learn how to moderate your animal and sensorial desires.

After studying and teaching traditional Far Eastern medicine and philosophy for many years, and having observed how this "forbidden" medicine has cured thousands of desperate, abandoned, "incurable" patients, I have learned the secret of health and a magnificent life. Here, from my experience, is a list of important suggestions:

1. Eliminate sugar completely from your diet.
2. Learn that it is possible to live without being carnivorous.
3. Eat primarily whole grains, vegetables, beans, and sea vegetables—all as unrefined as possible.
4. Eat as little as possible of all other foods. Live by the principle of *vivere parvo*, which means: be detached from all that is not absolutely and immediately necessary. Eat and drink only the absolute minimum, remembering that quantity changes quality—and that individual needs are different.
5. Control liquid intake to a minimum.

Follow these instructions for one month or more. You will see the results for yourself.

Before leaving this subject I would like to repeat that industrialized, commercial sugar is totally unnecessary, man having lived without it for thousands of years. It exists only for pleasure, and pleasure, being ruled by our lower sensorial judgment, often lures us into great dangers.

Some people find meat delicious. Our civilization of abundance and abuse supplies us with much of it, and the nutritional theory in favor nowadays strongly recommends it. But in point of fact, meat and other animal proteins are not at all "absolutely necessary." One can live without them. All animals can produce proteins peculiar to their species, even when they lack a source of nitrogen—organic or inorganic. All are endowed with the ability to transmute carbon and oxygen into nitrogen.

If, in accordance with modern nutritional theories, we consume large amounts of animal protein, we lose the ability to produce for ourselves our own special proteins. This is a net loss of adaptability—in other words, a decrease in vitality and independence. In actuality, proteins are produced by the body with excess materials that might be otherwise useless, appearing in storage form as rapidly growing nails, warts, or skin, especially on the sole of the foot. Cancer is the storage of excess that explodes, and we will examine this phenomenon more deeply later on. But for now, let us return to a consideration of the civilized people who, being very learned, anxious, and defeatist, mobilize all the scientific and technical means at their disposal in order to destroy symptoms. They come to a tragic end, including that of their own existence.

Civilized man has lost his dynamic adaptability, his key to infinite freedom. He has unknowingly replaced it with the finite and conditional liberty that is also known as sensory satisfaction. This liberty of slaves or prisoners is enticingly but mistakenly called comfort, pleasure, or high standard of living. Herein lies the largest defect in modern democracy. It is the crime of mechanical civilization.

Categories of Cure

According to my theory, there are three categories of cure:

1. Symptomatic: Elimination and destruction of symptoms by symptomatic methods—palliative, physical, violent cure. This is symptomatic, animal, or mechanical medicine.
2. Educational: Improvement of judgment to enable man to establish and maintain personal control of his physical health. This is the medicine of man.
3. Creative, Spiritual: A life without fear or anxiety, a life of freedom, happiness, and justice—the realization of self. This is the medicine of the body, the mind, and the soul.

If you are not certain that you want the third category of cure, by and for yourself and at any price, you have no need to study this book. You can find a temporary cure in the first category through popular, orthodox, or folk medicine; one in the second category can be achieved through some spiritual or psychological method. The third category, however, is the everlasting way that rises above the failures of the other two.

For a third-category cure, start with this part of my natural medicine that I offer to you freely:

1. Do not eat too much yin (expansive) food, that which diminishes or neutralizes the sodium content in your body. In a word, take only small amounts of water, very little fruit, and little salad.
2. Do not eat or drink anything that damages your basic physical quality or destroys your energy—for example: vinegar, all sugary foods, nightshades, coffee, chocolate or pastries, soft drinks—for a period of at least one month.
3. Brown rice, millet, buckwheat, and all the various unrefined grains should constitute at least 50 to 60 percent of your total diet.

That is all. It is very simple and yet it will guarantee you a big step on the way to self-improvement—good health, prevention of illness, and the preservation of your youthfulness. This is the unknown and very simple medicine completely simplified for your practice. Try it for one month. You will already be able to verify the results. It is the first practical lesson for curing all present or future illness by means of my macrobiotic method. And it costs you almost nothing.

Meats, animal protein, butter, cheese, fish, animal fat, and all animal products are completely unnecessary for maintaining your health; these products, as well as all other manufactured and modern industrial products, may be eliminated completely from your daily diet in order to re-establish or stabilize your physical condition and to develop and fortify your adaptability, imagination, memory, and judgment.

NO INCURABLE DISEASE

Incurable disease in man is a misnomer and a product of the

Wonder of Wonders

For many years, Shayne and I had both searched for a new way of life since we were generally unfulfilled and unhappy. She was particularly and constantly troubled by the fact that she had never been pregnant, despite nineteen years of examination and treatment by endless doctors.

In September of 1961, shortly after having been discharged by our then current psychotherapist (whether he felt that we had had enough help or that we were beyond help is still undetermined), we heard about what we considered to be a "silly" rice diet. Only as the result of a dare did we go to hear George Ohsawa speak at the Buddhist Academy in New York City. The outcome was that the skeptical Oleses dashed home as soon as the lecture was over to empty the refrigerator and cupboards of all non-macrobiotic foods. We had been convinced and were certain that if this man with the wonderfully deep voice were only 50 percent right about living and eating, we stood to gain the world.

About three weeks later, while transporting Mr. Ohsawa to a lecture on Long Island, Shayne broached the question of pregnancy to him. After inquiring at length about her likes and dislikes in relation to food and drink and about her mother and her tastes in food, he stated flatly that Shayne was not merely capable of having children but that she could become pregnant at will if she would only give up her highly yin diet. He said, "Eat 100-percent whole grains with a little gomashio, soy sauce, and drink strong mu tea." In his opinion, she had conceived hundreds of times in the past but had destroyed the newly-joined egg and sperm by means of a very yin diet consisting of much sugar, fruit, tomatoes, spices, and coffee.

She followed his instructions faithfully and, wonder of wonders, Shayne was pregnant one month later! Ohsawa had been right.

Lou Oles
Former editor of Ohsawa's writings

imagination. I have seen thousands of incurable diseases such as asthma, diabetes, epilepsy, leprosy, and paralyses of all kinds cured by macrobiotic practice in ten days or a few weeks. I am convinced that there is no incurable disease in all the world if we apply this method correctly.

No matter what method we use in the attempt to overcome sickness, we must first of all have a strong will to cure. This is particularly true for the macrobiotic way since here the individual must cure himself by himself and for himself, through his own comprehension of what is the true cause of his suffering.

We must be filled with the belief that our sickness can and will be cured through macrobiotic practice. This is neither a rigid, mystical, religious, unfounded belief nor a blind superstition. It is, rather, deepest understanding—the realization that justifiably and by all that is right, macrobiotic practice should cure illness for us because it has done just that for thousands of years in the Far East. It has simply and practically taught what is righteous food and natural living. It has inevitably led towards health, beauty, wisdom, and happiness.

I do not say dogmatically that those who believe in macrobiotic philosophy will be cured while the nonbelievers will suffer. I merely say that if it is not too late for a real cure, macrobiotic practice will achieve one because it is the way of nature.

I believe that illness is the crystallization of an error in our judgment, the tangible sign of a lack of natural orderliness in our lives. In allowing this condition to arise, either through poor thinking, ignorance, or apathy, we have done something wrong. To be healthy again, we must make a change—we must do something right. We must re-establish the orderly kind of existence that underlies and guarantees health.

By macrobiotic living, you undertake the rewarding task of putting your life in order, starting from its most basic point—eating and drinking. Righteous food is the materialization of God. God is revealed to us in it and by means of it. Our body—converted food—thus constitutes a speck of God Himself. The very reason that we can even live in this universe is that we are a speck of Him. And the reason that this speck becomes sick or unhappy is that it forgets its origin; it loses sight of the totality of which it is a minute part.

If we know God or wholeness and at the same time are deeply aware of our own personal "speckness," we cannot avoid being beautiful, healthy, wise, and happy. To realize this and then to live with that realization as our motivation is macrobiotic living.

The will to cure is vastly different from the impulse to escape from the symptoms of a disease, an urge prompted by pain and suffering. The person who seeks a palliative or pain-killer, who believes that his salvation lies in the right kind of surgery or in finding the right doctor, is motivated by short-sighted, wishful thinking—not will. True will is the relentless drive to discover the law of life—the origin, mechanism, structure, value, and end of justice. If this is what stirs you to action, then all your ills are curable.

You must be able to say:

I will cure my sickness. I will live in justice; I will live in God.

I am fearful and sick because I have violated the law of nature. To discover and correct this violation is more vital to my existence than the cure itself.

If I understand righteous macrobiotic practice—the materialization of the law of nature—my sickness must be cured.

If I cannot cure myself, then both my understanding and my way of making the law of nature a practical part of my life are superficial.

I must study more deeply.

This is the will to cure.

WHEN WILL YOU BE CURED?

When will you be cured? I often answer, "You will be cured in ten days to two months." And yet you do not find yourself cured within that period. Why? I have stated repeatedly that macrobiotic living cures all diseases within ten days, that it changes the body's orientation toward health, away from disease. Disease is the exact barometer of our mistakes, of our abuse, of our ignorance of the

Curing With Whiskey

*When Ohsawa lectured at the Wurtsboro Summer Camp in the Cat-
skill Mountains in 1961, he was already acquainted with English so
he was giving lectures more freely and without much preparation.
Also, he was experimenting on himself concerning the physical effect
of yogurt.*

*One Sunday, he asked me, "Herman, could you please get me a
bottle of whiskey."*

*"It is Sunday, there is no liquor store open," I told him while
wondering why he wanted whiskey.*

*"But I need it today," he replied sternly. The sense of urgency in
his voice prompted me to find some. I went to the camp manager's home
and borrowed from him.*

*It wasn't until later that I learned that Ohsawa had severe pain in
his stomach from the yogurt experiments and the whiskey enabled him to
give his lecture without noticing the pain. For Ohsawa, sickness was a
game and he was very good at figuring out how to win the game.*

Herman Aihara
Founder of the George Ohsawa Macrobiotic Foundation
and Vega Study Center

Order of the Universe. It is therefore said that there can be no cure
unless we recognize our own faults, our own ignorance, and,
above all, the Order of the Universe, the key to our health, freedom, and justice. But what is justice? Everyone thinks he knows,
but in reality ...

According to Far Eastern philosophy justice is absolute, infinite,
eternal, and universal—a larger concept, by far, than that of Western justice. The commonly understood meaning of justice is relative,
personal, finite, and conditional. Democratic justice as defined by
John Locke is only known by the majority. In actuality, there is no

single concept in Western thought that is the equivalent of the Far Eastern concept of justice. Justice is another name for happiness that is infinite and eternal. A macrobiotic individual is a student of the way to such infinite happiness. The Unifying Principle or, in other words, life itself, is the only teacher of this all-embracing justice.

Most of you look for a rapid cure, and make large statements about your willingness to pay any price to achieve it. Still, you only attempt to understand basic yin-yang functioning where it concerns your immediate diet. Worse yet, you allow others to tell you what to eat. You abandon all pursuit of the Unifying Principle as soon as your physical difficulties have disappeared. In short, the patient is never willing to pay the true price.

Two persons come to mind, both of whom were not completely cured by macrobiotic practice. In each case, their sickness returned. Neither could understand that disease cannot leave the patient entirely until he discovers and acknowledges his own mistakes. So many individuals are relieved of their anxieties and suffering by following a macrobiotic diet, yet become ill again because they do not probe even deeper into the Unifying Principle, the law of life.

I have understood, once and for all, that one must not cure anyone else. Everyone must do it for himself, by himself. If your wish is to gain a reputation, to have a good income, to enjoy a sentimental self-esteem, then you can, of course, make a career of taking care of people.

When will you be cured? In ten days, most assuredly, if you sincerely admit to yourself your own mistakes. The kind of disease makes no difference, since all diseases are a variation of man's loss of balance—biological, psychological, or spiritual. If you are not cured in ten days or two months, you have no right to criticize my teaching. You have only to regret your own poor understanding of infinite and absolute justice.

WHAT WE MUST NOT CURE

No disease is incurable for God, Creator of this infinite universe— the kingdom of freedom, happiness, and justice. Nevertheless, there are some sick people who cannot be cured, and who cannot be taught to cure themselves. They are the arrogant ones who do not wish to know first of all the structure of the infinite universe and its Unifying Principle (the kingdom of heaven and its justice). They do not realize that without this knowledge they cannot have the faith that orders the mountain to enter the sea.

If you do not have the will to live most simply and happily, you must not and cannot be cured.

Sick people incessantly express the wish for a cure; they claim to have the will to rid themselves of disease at any cost. Will of this variety is merely a desire to escape from the status quo—defeatism. It reveals an unwillingness to accept the eternal order in life, the order that oscillates between difficulty and pleasure. To exist in a static state that includes only the one and not the other is impossible: we must continually re-create our own happiness by recognizing and curing disease at every instant of our lives.

Many a man wishes to be cured by others or by some mechanical device, all the while bypassing his own involvement and personal responsibility, the cause of his disease: mea culpa . . . my crime. People of this sort are descendants of the race of vipers. They do not deserve a complete cure or the kingdom of heaven. They must not and, in fact, cannot be cured.

True will, by contrast, is unique and works in quite a different manner. The true will to live seeks and finds, first of all, the fundamental cause of all unhappiness, all disease, all injustice in the world and then proceeds to eliminate it without using violent, artificial means. It conquers through methods that are in accord with the structure of the infinite universe, naturally and peacefully.

The drive to cure only symptoms or to have control of one's health without accepting responsibility is comparable to the notion on the part of an individual that he can step in front of a moving train and not be struck down. It is simple exclusiveness and egoism; it eclipses and denies true will, the Order of the Universe.

CANCER: THE MOST DREADED ENEMY

And, then, there is cancer.

Civilized people consider this disease a natural phenomenon and the most terrible curse to which human society has ever been subjected. Such a fear-crazed attitude is exclusive, lonely, and egocentric, signifying a closed mind and a rigid body, and resembles the behavior of a little cat, his back humped and his hair erect before a vicious dog. Such fear (the front) and hostility (the back) become greater and greater and are nourished at the same source. They are Siamese twins sharing the same heart.

"Cancer is the most dreadful enemy in the history of mankind."

This exclusive and arrogant statement completely negates the Christian principle, "Do not resist, not even evil." But cancer is not your neighbor, or even a tenant in your house. Cancer is indeed your blood-brother. To react with hostility is to admit fear. Hostility and fear are characteristic of a man who lacks confidence, universal love, and generosity, who is already beaten and defeated. The therapeutics of symptomatic medicine is the corollary of this defeatist mentality.

In order to cure a cancer patient who has already surrendered, it is first necessary to change his attitude. This must be accomplished at any cost. Otherwise, everything is useless and the patient might just as well be dead.

People in more primitive cultures who study and apply the dialectical monistic philosophy are also surprised at the appearance of cancer. But they feel neither fear nor hostility. Instead they react as would a cheerful, smiling, innocent child who has been given so much to be thankful for. He is sorry to have caused so much trouble. Such is the response of noncivilized people toward their universal father, Tao: the Order of the Universe. When scolded with cancer, they examine themselves very deeply in order to discover what they have done to deserve this reprimand. They understand that nothing unpleasant or sorrowful is needlessly produced, but that on the contrary, all that is given is necessary, useful, or agreeable: food, drink, sun, moon, stars, mountains, fresh air, water, fish, flowers, atoms, infinite space and time. All this is given freely. How can we not accept all with the deepest gratitude? What fools we are to protest.

A man of sensory judgment is a slave to his tastes. His condition is fraught with danger. The decline of world empires, as well as that of any organism, begins from within. Only fearful, exclusive, defeatist, and irresponsible people claim that unhappiness comes from the outside, thus revealing their dependence on external conditions, their state of voluntary slavery. He who accuses another stands accused himself (of his dependence on the other).

The Order of the Universe, which sustains, animates, destroys, and transmutes everything, the visible and the invisible, is absolute justice. All who are not aware of this absolute justice must pay a high price.

All functions develop through being exercised, and protein-storage, which eventuates in cancer, is no exception. It stands to reason that the more one partakes of needless proteins, the more efficient this storage mechanism will become.

Protein is provided to the body's internal environment by the blood, and blood is manufactured in the intestines from digested food particles. I arrived at this conviction of many years' standing through an application of the incomparable Unifying Principle. In recent years, Professors Chishima and Morishita of Japan succeeded in microscopically filming the transformation of digested food particles into blood, and that of red cells into proteinic cancer elements, scientifically substantiating my position and clearly disproving the hypothesis that blood is manufactured in bone marrow—an hypothesis arrived at by observing the change in bone marrow in the blood of sick people.

The mechanisms that transform digested food particles into blood, and blood into cancer cells, are yin. Both of these transformations can be reversed at will by one who knows how to apply yang factors.

But what is cancer?

Cancer does not grow old, it does not fall ill; it develops, stops, sleeps, awakens, and resumes its activities. It repeats such cycles indefinitely. It resists, adapts. triumphs. It is life itself. It is blind, mechanical will, that is to say insatibility, voracity, uncontrolled growth. It is therefore unbalanced. Too much of the material and not enough of the non-material. Why this disharmony between matter and spirit? Everything has a cause.

The cause of cancer is dualistic, materialistic man. He is like King Midas who, in realizing his most cherished dream, changed everything into gold. Modern Midas attempts to organize the world toward satisfaction of his blind and sensory desires, and the result is cancer, which grows blindly and indefinitely, responsive to the destructive touch of a humanity that has abandoned its soul in favor of the Cartesian or Aristotelian dichotomy. Quantity changes quality. King Midas has lost his perspective and with it his bearing. He no longer perceives, and can no longer find, meaning in superabundant matter. Rather he has found the opposite: uncertainty, fear, anguish, war, and burgeoning cancer.

Now, he must listen, if he can still hear. Let him only acknowledge the voice of the non-materialistic, metaphysical, moral civilization that lives in cooperation with nature by consciously applying the principles and theorems of the Order of the Universe and its practical application of the Unifying Principle, and his perspective will return once more.

Cancer is a most interesting malady. It is considered, along with heart and mental disease, one of the three most destructive scourges of our time, a striking illustration of the ineffectiveness of modern symptomatic medicine.

Lack of understanding of the structure of the infinite universe and its order makes it impossible for modern medicine to cure even an insignificant wart, and what is more important, to prevent its occurrence in the first place. All symptomatic treatment is analytical and consequently prohibitive, negative, and destructive. For example, it attempts to lower fever without knowing the origin and mechanism of the fever; it uses antibiotics against all microbial diseases without eliminating that which makes microbes dangerous; finally, it destroys suffering organs through surgery without dealing with the real cause of disease: man's faulty judgment in eating and drinking.

Cancer, mental disease, and cardiac ailments are simply the result, the dead-end of symptomatic medicine, which does not comprehend the life process itself. Cancer is the most extreme yin disease. However, no illness is more simple to cure than cancer (this also applies to mental disease and heart trouble) through a return to the most elementary and natural eating and drinking.

Individual differences with regard to natural immunity to cancer must be explained. Even more importantly, we must be clearly told what natural immunity is. Neither modern medicine nor physiology provides an answer, but instead camouflages ignorance with meaningless terminology. Immunity is "something unknown and incomprehensible"—a worthy counterpart of the "feverish humors" of Molière's medical comedies.

Immunity (resistance to any potential sickness) is a characteristic of health, according to the practical, dialectical philosophy of the Far East. And what is health? It is the normal condition of all living beings. And what is life? As will be shown in Chapter 6 on the Order of the Universe, it is the materialization of the invisible infinite through extended stages of cosmogonic, energetic, nuclear, and atomic organization, followed by geological eras of monocellular and multicellular organization that culminates in man. Inversely, it is the lengthy return trip through dematerialization towards eternal spiritualization.

LIFE'S ART

I have given you a very brief sketch of Far Eastern medicine. The first step for you is to try my preparatory dietetic instructions for the sick. I repeat them:

1. Do not eat white sugar and avoid everything that is sugared.
2. Look for the minimum quantity of water that is necessary to your existence and that will require you to urinate no more than three to four times per day.
3. Use the least possible amount of animal products, especially if you reside in a warm climate or if you are going to visit one.

4. Avoid industrial foods, particularly those colored with dye-stuff.

5. Avoid foods imported from afar. A free trade economy violates the laws of the universe in our diet and consequently undermines our health.

6. Avoid potatoes, tomatoes, eggplant, and fruit in the case of yin sickness.

7. Do not eat vinegar.

8. Include in your diet 50 to 60 percent whole grains and 20 to 25 percent well-cooked or baked vegetables.

9. Prepare food by any traditional method.

10. Chew food as thoroughly as possible, an average of about fifty times each mouthful.

In proportion to the improvement of your constitution, you will also improve in yin-yang discrimination, and as your judgment improves, you will catch sight of new horizons of traditional Far Eastern medicine.

If you should decide to study my five-thousand-year-old philosophy in order to realize infinite freedom, eternal happiness, and absolute righteousness, understand that you must do this on your own, independently, by and for yourself, as do all animals, birds, insects, and fish. First of all, make up your mind to conquer your sickness—not his or hers, but yours.

Learn the nature of your disease and its cause. If you are only interested in the disappearance of symptoms, difficulties, or pain, you have no need to study this book. This unique philosophy does not deal with symptomatic medicine.

To assimilate and understand the Unifying Principle thoroughly, you must live it in your daily life by observing a macrobiotic diet. You yourself can be the creator of your own life, health, and happiness.

Occasionally, after having listened to the list of foods that are to be avoided, someone asks: "But what, then, *can* we eat?" The one who asks is simple-minded, egocentric, and too fond of his taste. Here is the true reason for his illness and misfortune. It is

Unlocking the Door

*I first met George Ohsawa in 1959 at a lecture in New York City. My
father had lung cancer, and I asked Ohsawa how I could help my dad.
Ohsawa looked at me and said, "You cannot help anybody until you help
yourself. You have an enlarged heart and should avoid vitamin C for three
years." Then he turned away from me. I got so mad that I ate only whole
grains for a whole week and to my surprise this cured my lifelong sinus
condition. It changed my life completely.*

*Many times, I heard Ohsawa say, "I can only give you the keys,
you must unlock the door. There are many doors, you must decide
which one to open."*

Dick Smith
Retired from Chico-San, Inc.

an involuntary acknowledgment of his egoism, of the original and
daily sin that he unconsciously commits. He does not know that
in every country of the world, with few exceptions, there are
natural foods by the hundreds and that a good cook can prepare
hundreds of delicious dishes in quite different ways, with the same
foods.

Culinary art is life's art. Our health and consequently our
happiness, our liberty, and even our judging ability are under
the influence of this art. This is why only the best disciples are
selected as cooks in the great schools or Buddhist convents. If
you are not a good cook, you simply have to learn the culinary
art.

Culinary preparation is, indeed, fundamental in enabling man
to attain self-realization through Far Eastern medicine. So-called
health and happiness or liberty and peace, the greatest edifices of
humanity, must be erected on a biological, physical, and logical
foundation: proper eating and drinking.

THE VIRUS

"Matter is non-matter and energy comes from nowhere."
    Nuclear science.
"Nonsense!" despaired Professor Bridgman
    Before taking his life.
    Visible and invisible, physical and metaphysical,
    Scientific medicine dreams it discovered the ultimate
    killer:
    The virus!
Ghost and nightmare, it deludes a world of
    Helpless doctors . . . fascinated, amazed, in despair.
But true humanity, turning its face from the microscope
    to the macrocosm
Will contemplate the limitless horizons of
The infinite universe
And owe to the virus a new medicine—
Fundamental and divine, full of life.
Ah! Universal understanding.

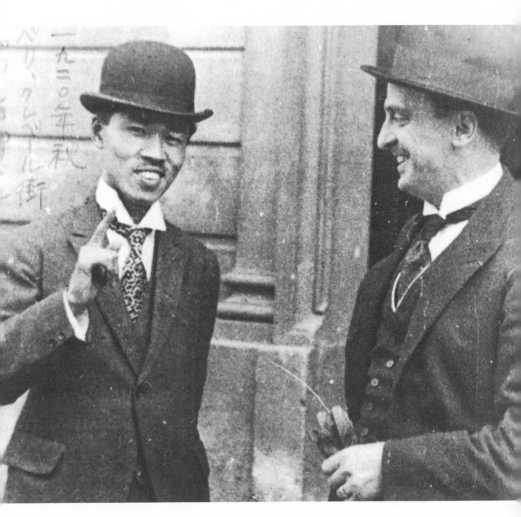

George Ohsawaw, age twenty-seven, in Paris, 1920.

Part Two

PRINCIPLES
OF THE MIND

Happiness or misery, health or sickness, freedom or slavery—
all depend upon the manner in which we conduct our daily lives
and activities. Our conduct is dictated by our judgment.
It, in turn, is a result of our comprehension of the structure
of the world and the infinite universe.

George Ohsawa
Zen Macrobiotics

4

JUDGING ABILITY

SEVEN STAGES OF JUDGMENT

Our happiness depends upon our judgment. Illness or health, intelligence or foolishness, piety or vice depend upon our judgment. Judgment develops upward toward perfection, in the way I show below, from one to seven.

1. Physical judgment (mechanical and blind).
2. Sensorial judgment (pleasant and unpleasant).
3. Sentimental judgment (what is desirable and undesirable).
4. Intellectual judgment (conceptual, scientific).
5. Social judgment (social reason's judgment: morals and economy).
6. Ideological judgment (religious thinking, justice and injustice).
7. Supreme judgment (absolute and universal love that embraces everything and turns every antagonism into complementarity).

At the time of birth and for some time thereafter, we are unable to form any judgment. Then the physical judgment, the lowest one, awakens.

After some days, the sensorial judgment begins to function and to perceive cold and warmth, two poles of our relative world. It develops from day to day, and gradually can distinguish all the degrees between two extremes: colors, shapes, temperatures, agreeable or disagreeable tastes, sympathy or hostility. This latter stage of development occurs within a few weeks.

After some months, we reach the affective emotional, sentimental judgment. We discern what attracts us affectively and what frightens us or may harm us, etc.

In the fourth stage, judgment develops in us the true concept of the two antagonistic categories: good and evil, beautiful and ugly, useful and useless, healthy food and poison, just and unjust. This intellectual stage also includes all natural or scientific categories.

On reaching the fifth stage, judgment turns social and perceives a wider horizon: economy and morality.

In the sixth stage, ideology develops (dualism, materialism, spiritualism, life's affirmation or negation, etc.).

It is in the seventh stage, the very last one, that our judging ability reaches the constitution of the universe and life, where we are able to embrace all opposites in order to establish the grand universal unification.

Such is, in my opinion, a general sketch of the natural development of our judgment. It is innate and can be likened to memory, the basis of our faculty for adaptation, and its expansion is but our self-realization (or the realization of life itself). This realization can be destroyed, deformed, and repressed under the influence of the biological, physiological, and social surroundings during childhood. It is then the beginnings of our misfortune and the reason why some souls are detained and remain behind. Their judging remains childish and undeveloped. This is the case with all those who look toward symptomatic medicine and all those who love wealth, strength, and authority—such as famous politicians, industrialists, soldiers, physicians, etc. Of course, they are not entirely responsible for this state of mind; their surroundings are greatly responsible, for they impede and stop the natural and total development of judgment.

Table 4.1 classifies the origins of man's thoughts and actions according to the seven stages of judgment.

The first four stages of this evolution are egocentric. A great many people who consider themselves pacifists are, in fact, sentimental and simplistic, for their judging belongs only to the third stage. Real pacifists and peacemakers must possess the seventh stage of judgment. Most pacifists are those who do not like war; they are afraid of war, and this is the reason for their pacifism. They are not aware of war's origin, and without being aware of its origin, one cannot solve a problem. One need not be afraid of war, but one must perceive one's own egoism, one's sentimentality and lack of fortitude, which can be one cause of war. This is true for all of us, large and small, philanthropic and religious, if we do not live according to the *vivere parvo* principle: eat and drink only what is necessary.

In any case, one cannot possess supreme judging ability (the seventh stage of judgment) from the very beginning. One must first develop the lowest judgment. Therefore, one must endure heat, cold, hunger, and the greatest difficulties, not only in childhood, but all during one's entire life (*vivere parvo*). And as one grows older, life seems more agitated and full of difficulties and sadness. One must love and be betrayed.

Without having lived such a life, one cannot and must not unfold one's conceptual faculty of judgment. Later, the judging ability expands, through social and ideological life, to the supreme ability. And the supreme judging ability must be strengthened, developed, and increased infinitely by training the lower categories of judgment at the same time as the higher ones, since "the greater and wider the back, the greater and wider the front." The seven stages of judgment are not alien to and independent of each other, but just different degrees of the same judging ability. They are the roots, trunk, boughs, foliage, flowers, and fruit of this "judgment tree." In order for boughs to develop and for flowers and fruit to be produced in large quantities under a fine sky, there must be thick and thin roots reaching deep into rich black soil.

Table 4.1 Classification of the Stages of Human Development

Stage of Judgment	Learning	Love	Profession	Eating and Drinking
7th Supreme	Self-realization, illumination, tao, satori	All-embracing	Happy man, fulfills all his dreams throughout life	Eats and drinks anything with great pleasure
6th Ideological	Philosophy, religion, dialectics	Spiritual	Thinker, originator of theories	Follows dietetic or religious principle
5th Social	Economics, morality	Social	Organizer	Conformist—like everyone else
4th Intellectual	Science, arts	Understanding, scientific, systematic, calculating, expert	Wholesaler of knowledge and techniques	According to a theory of nutrition
3rd Sentimental	Literature	Emotionally universal	Wholesaler of emotions	Gourmet (connoisseur)
2nd Sensory	Dance, gymnastics, conditioned reflexes	Erotic, seeking physical comfort and sensual pleasure	Wholesaler of pleasure: actor, merchant, novelist, prostitute	Gourmand (greedy eater)
1st Physical	Instinctive or unconscious reflexes	Instinctive (appetite, hunger)	He who sells his life—working slave, salaried employee	Guided only by hunger and thirst

CURING THE SICK

Macrobiotic practice can cure disease symptoms easily. The difficulty lies in curing the patient. He must learn how to unfetter himself, cast off his shackles, and walk upright, unafraid, a natural man, a free man. But learning to be free requires the total involvement of heart, imagination, faith, and will.

The technique for curing sickness is called medicine. To cure, one must know the cause of sickness. However, modern medicine does not know the cause. What modern medicine calls cause is merely symptoms, or the results of sickness. The reason modern medicine cannot cure so many diseases lies in the fact that it does not know the cause of disease.

Then what is the cause of disease? In my opinion, the cause of disease is the condition in which one's supreme judging ability is clouded or eclipsed. All animals other than man have lower judging ability only, which is the first, second, and third stages of judgment, and are lacking the fourth, fifth, and sixth stages of judgment. Therefore, they reveal the supreme judging ability more easily than man. In the case of man, who has the fourth through sixth stages of judgment, the supreme judging ability is eclipsed. But why do the fourth, fifth, and sixth stages of judgment eclipse the seventh stage of judgment or the supreme judging ability?

Judgment is a compass giving us directions and decisions in our travels through life. One who makes a wrong judgment goes the wrong direction, and the result is unhappiness or sickness. Sickness is the first warning that we have made a wrong judgment. A healthy person is never unhappy. If he is, his health is only physical, not total and real health; or his health is "given" health from parents or others.

For example, we may analyze a painting by the amount, quality, and cost of color used. But by improving these, we can never improve the picture. The skill of the painter must be improved. For that, his thinking, idea, or concept of life must be improved. Modern medicine tries to cure sickness by analyzing the color. It is completely forgetting the painter, who uses the color and designs the picture.

Second Birth

When my sister met George Ohsawa in London, he immediately said upon hearing her name, "I want to meet your father in Belgium to talk about World Government as we are both leaders in this movement."

Ohsawa came to our house and, without anyone's telling him, guessed that I had an "incurable" bone illness. He gave me the necessary instructions to get better and after four days, all the pain was gone. I was totally cured after two months and resumed my agricultural activities that I had stopped one year before.

Although I was well, I thought I could get even better by restricting my diet more. I even stopped drinking liquid. Harvesting grains by hand was very hard work and my legs became heavy. A few days later, instead of three urinations a day, I had more than ten. One evening as I was almost dying, my sister phoned Ohsawa while we were meeting with doctors in Paris.

"Give him two liters of cooked rice water immediately," was Ohsawa's response. Later that evening, he told the doctors, "Probably too late, Pierre will die. Bad judgment, he does what I write instead of using his own judgment."

That evening was my second birth and the beginning of my true understanding of the Order of the Universe.

Pierre Gevaert
Founder of the LIMA Company

Most medicine aims at curing symptoms. When it realizes that the symptomatic cure is useless or endless or dangerous, it turns to other ways. One of them is psychic, psychological, and religious healing, and the other one is social and preventive medicine. However, these also tend to be symptomatic cures. Macrobiotic medicine aims at curing man, and not sickness only, because man is the producer of sickness. Without curing man, no sickness is cured.

We can see how emphasis on the fourth, fifth, and sixth stages of development helps to eclipse the seventh or supreme stage.

Western medicine must develop to be a preventive medicine. Preventive medicine must develop into the way of health—macrobiotic philosophy. The way of health must reach to a way of living. The principle of such a way of living must be simple and universal. Such a principle should not be a difficult and sophisticated concept, but must be an easy and practical one that can be applied by anyone in daily life.

Mastering macrobiotic medicine means becoming a man who devotes himself to the search of infinite freedom, eternal happiness, and absolute justice, and being a man who doesn't worry about money, power, knowledge, status, and fame. However skillful you are in any technique, you will be far from real freedom, happiness, and justice if your aim is money, status, or fame. This is true in the case of medicine. The more expensive the medicine becomes, the more unjust, unfree, and unhappy it becomes. Air cooled by an air-conditioner is more expensive and harmful to us than air in the woods. Sunlight is cheaper and healthier than any artificial light or radiation. Water from mountain streams without pollution is much cheaper and more health-giving than soda, factory-made orange juice, or beer.

All plants grow with only sunshine, air, and water, and they are beautiful, strong, and gentle. Animals are the same. The Angora rabbit of Peru has immunity to all bacterial diseases. This finding has made the animal important in medical study. It lives in the high mountains of Peru where sunlight is weak and air is thin. The secret of its immunity is that it doesn't drink much. It drinks only for necessity. Excess water makes the blood thin, which in turn weakens the immune power and also thins nutrition, weakening the heart and kidneys as a result. In short, excessive and greedy eating and drinking are the cause of all sicknesses. True medicine must be cheap; it can be acquired any place at any time.

Lao-tsu said, "Winning without weapons is the real winning." Macrobiotic medicine is a medicine without weapons such as knives, needles, drugs, chemicals, and radiation. Macrobiotic medicine is a teaching of awareness of the reality or the Order of the Universe through sickness. In this sense, macrobiotic medicine is more religious than modern religions. In fact, macrobiotic people acquire real religion, and not superstitions. In other words, when you realize that you are the cause of the sickness and that sickness is the benefactor of your life; when you like everyone and reach the mentality of Will Rogers who said, "I never met a man I didn't like"; and when you appreciate anything including sickness, misfortune, and difficulties; then you graduate from macrobiotic medicine. To reach this state of mind, I recommend the following practical method:

- Eat whole grains and local, seasonal vegetables, using a bit of salt, oil, and traditional condiments.
- Chew each mouthful of food fifty times or more.
- Drink only what is necessary.
- Work hard physically.

After three years of observing the above diet and way of living, you can firmly establish health. After that, teach macrobiotic living to others for seven years. Then, devote yourself to whatever you want most in your life.

HEALING POWER OF THE MIND

I am convinced that a sick man is a criminal and that sickness is his punishment. Small children are exceptions since they are not old enough to judge for themselves. Their punishment is meted out instead to their parents in the form of the anguish they suffer when the children are ill.

Anyone who becomes ill or has ailing children knows neither God nor the Order of the Universe.

Our bodies—knowable, seeable, touchable—are part of and bound to this relative, material world. Our minds, by contrast, are absolutely free to go anywhere at any time in the absolute, infinite world. We have the power to look into the past or future in an instant.

The world of mind is in reality the world of God; it is infinity or oneness. Since all of us possess a mind, we are inhabitants without choice of the absolute world of God. We cannot say, in all honesty, that we do not know it. He who says, "I do not know God," or who behaves as if he does not know Him, is the biggest criminal of all. Compared with him, all other offenders are petty.

He who cannot live in the infinite world—the world of mind—will never be happy or achieve anything of real worth. He always ends in sickness and sorrow.

Epictetus has said, "Of all the things to be known, there is only one that is worth classifying as either good or bad. To know or acknowledge God or infinity is a good thing. Not to know or acknowledge either one is bad. The consideration of good or bad in reference to all other things is by comparison insignificant and inconsequential. It is the product of a superficial concept of the world."

In macrobiotic thinking, we say that sickness comes from food. This can be proven to be true. Our choice of food, however, is actually determined by the mind. If we know God, or mind, we never choose bad food. He who does not know God and cannot see the Order of the Universe cannot find the right food and becomes sick. Physical illness is an indication of illness of mind or illness in thinking.

Mind and God being one and the same, it is easy to see that what overcomes illness is mind. If one does not enter this world of mind, one can neither cure disease nor be happy. In the Far East, mind means absolute or Tao or discipline. In this light, it is understandable that for God it is not difficult to cure sickness and unhappiness.

Since in macrobiotic thinking we understand that sickness of character or mind is caused by food, we naturally feel that its cure as well is rooted in food. From this fundamental point, it is a simple thing to eliminate physical illness.

He who thinks that macrobiotic living is merely a cure for physical ailments, however, can never really be helped. It is not a new medicine to stop pain or suffering, but rather a teaching that goes to the source of pain and eradicates it. Once this kind of cure has been effected, the disease will never recur. Consequently, macrobiotic consultation is given once in a lifetime. I consult with an individual one time; those who return again indicate that they have never sought out the true cause of their difficulty.

Some people think that macrobiotic philosophy is no more than the teaching of a diet—the eating of brown rice, carrots, and gomashio (sesame salt). Others imagine that it is summed up in the statement, "Don't eat cake and sugar." How far from the truth!

Macrobiotic living is the process of changing ourselves so that we can eat anything we like without fear of becoming ill; it enables us to live a joyful life during which we can achieve anything we choose. It is knowing the infinite, giving thanks to the infinite, and always having a feeling of wonder and gratefulness towards the infinite. Without this, we do not have real health; our lives are spent in the contemplation of suffering and trouble.

Should an individual happen to have physical health alone, without being on intimate terms with the infinite, he will never feel great joy or security. If he observes the macrobiotic way of life, however, he will inevitably acquire the mentality with which to live a happy life, in peace always.

The person who has never been sick is not truly secure, because his health is a gift from his parents. They have provided him with a strong foundation that he can eventually destroy through bad judgment.

True health is that which you yourself have created out of illness. Only if you have produced your own health can you know how wonderful it actually is. For this reason, many healthy people squander away their health; through ignorance, they spoil it without knowing its true value. He who knows the real worth of health spreads his joyous knowledge by telling others what he knows. If you are healthy but do not try to give to others of the happiness it brings, you are unaware that happiness is priceless.

The aim of macrobiotic philosophy is to provide the means for establishing a joyful attitude. In the face of it, all arrogance, complaints, fear, insecurity, sadness, and suffering fade into nothingness. Happiness, love, freedom, and faith remain. In such a state there is infinite gratitude.

George Saved My Life

I became a pilot in World War II. The United States had reached Okinawa and we were sent to the south of Kyushu where we would take off to attack the Americans. We would bomb them at night and return to Kyushu by morning.

Then in April of 1945, I received a letter from George Ohsawa. He was in jail in Niigata Prefecture. "Your condition is very yang," he wrote, "so be careful. Very dangerous." He could tell from my letters to him, from my handwriting.

"You must become more yin," he wrote, "try fasting, don't eat anything for one week." He said this so I would become too weak to fly. He sent letters like that to about sixty of his students who were also pilots.

But our squadron commander wanted us to make another nighttime attack on Okinawa. I told him, "I cannot fly at nighttime to Okinawa. I don't have the strength to fly for five hours."

They never came back. After five days, only the major returned. If it hadn't been for George, maybe I would have died.

Junsei Yamazaki (Yagi)
Producer of macrobiotic products

We give thanks to and for everything. The man who is at this level radiates gratitude; his world is full. Even if he becomes ill or has great difficulty, such a man can change his suffering into happiness immediately. If someone attacks him with a stone, that stone changes into a flower; if the weapon is a sword, the sword becomes a mirror. If he is given poison, the poison is medicine.

Macrobiotic philosophy teaches us to translate this ephemeral, narrow, relative, sad, unfree world into an infinitely joyful heaven.

If you have neither the intention to understand nor the desire to enter this seventh heaven, you had better not be macrobiotic. He who does not want to enter the seventh heaven has the biggest sickness of all—egoism. He is no better than those who seek only fame, wealth, or position. Here is the biggest crime—the foundation of all unhappiness. What greater unhappiness can there be than to think, "Now I am rich" or "I have nothing to worry about—I am healthy." Wealth or health of this variety can change to poverty or sickness overnight.

Macrobiotic living is as necessary for healthy people as it is for the sick; in fact, the so-called healthy ones must be helped first. But since they are usually content with their small good fortune and are not seeking anything more, they are difficult to reach. People who are suffering are easily helped because they have pain as a reason to seek health.

He who is sick and yet understands infinity is much happier than he who is healthy but cannot enter seventh heaven. I am thus grateful for illness.

Modern medicine cures the symptoms of illness by artificial means such as an injection or a pill; the patient's understanding never enters into the whole process. Those treated in this manner lose their chance to enter the kingdom of heaven. I believe that modern medicine does man a great injustice in this way.

Healing power is in our minds. The material for opening our minds and for healing disease, however, is food, the qualities of which we distinguish through our minds. If we cannot clear our minds, we cannot distinguish correct food. Healing power is in the mind. Sickness is given to us so that we may discover this mind. If we cannot, we had better remain ill until we do. This is the order of God.

However, we must be grateful to modern medicine. Through the suffering it gives us, we have the motivation to change, to understand God and the Order of the Universe. We are thus given the opportunity to achieve the fullest health and happiness.

THE MOST COMPLETE EDUCATION OF ALL

The Fundamental Basis of All Education

Modern education is scientific. Its ideal is the extension of understanding through data derived from the senses—second stage

Childlike Education

I fondly remember a meeting arranged by Françoise Rivière at the Paris Ignoramus Center with Renè Levy, a French macrobiotic teacher still active today, and Jiro Nakamura, who directed the Ohsawa House in Germany. The discussion centered on the special power that George Ohsawa used to galvanize and captivate the children in his audiences. Was it the pure, joyous spirit that was always evident in his lectures here as well as abroad? Could it be his genuine love for the very young or his very original style of delivery combined with his superb show-manship?

*We concluded, it was mostly due to the element of surprise. Mr. Ohsawa would unexpectedly point at someone in the audience and demand an immediate answer, then move rapidly to someone else if the first did not respond fast enough. Invariably, the children present were delighted since quite often they would have the answer well before their parents could even begin to formulate an answer. The solution offered by a child was simple, crystal clear, and exemplary based on the simplest logic and an intuitive understanding of the Unifying Principle. Laughing at the cumbersome and impractical solution offered by the adults, George would point out that if children invariably had the right answer, we would do well to acquire the same child-like approach to the world's problems. (One of Mr. Ohsawa's favorite children's books was St. Exupery's *The Little Prince*.)*

What Levy observed during that Paris meeting is that an audience that is constantly invited to participate and fails in thinking with originality and simplicity, is going to be motivated to study much harder after the lectures. At Ohsawa's macrobiotic camps around the world, the conversations during and long after dinner were most lively and centered less on the origin or the quality of the food served and more on the topics and the challenges of the lectures. Ohsawa moti-vated countless people in this way.

Jacques de Langre
Founder of the Grain and Salt Society

judgment. This education has become professional and conformist technique.

The average American is no longer accustomed to thinking; he has become the victim of a "let-someone-else-do-it" push-button existence. Americans, educated in a manner that is too pragmatic and encyclopedic, are taught to be good professionals—machine-men or slaves. In the United States more than in any other country, I have been shocked by the number of people who cannot use their innate ability to judge. They have eyes and ears but they do not see or hear. They are only suspicious. They know only the relative, limited, and ephemeral world where nothing is constant; where happiness, freedom, and justice are short-lived.

In the beginning of the nineteenth century, modern education was founded on the idea that science creates superior conditions for human life. The great dream of science, then, is that one day what is regarded as the greatest of all calamities—unhappiness due to poverty—will be banished from the earth.

Traditional Far Eastern education, which originated five thousand years ago, was founded on a completely opposite idea from modern education. It taught that one should enjoy poverty and consider it a blessing; that one should regard difficulties and suffering with gratitude, as a help or guide; that a simple roof sufficed for shelter; and that a handful of whole rice and a few vegetables were sufficient as food.

It taught that one should consider cold and heat as teachers which fortify, rather than treat them as enemies; that it is not necessary to kill animals, and even less necessary to kill bacteria. It also taught that one should adapt oneself to everything and everyone, that one should treat others like a spring breeze while strengthening oneself with autumn frosts; that one should pardon others, respect others, and love everyone in the conviction that all is given inexhaustibly; that one should not hesitate to give one's life for others; that one should devote oneself to the search for truth—that is, the Unifying Principle—and to practice peace, purity, and respect for the principles underlying macrobiotic philosophy in daily life.

Education in the ancient Far East was profoundly spiritual, and taught that adaptation to nature is the way to arrive at the supreme state of judgment. Later, this was degraded by conformist and conceptual educators, who advocated a system that pretended to teach seeds and buds how to immediately become fruits and flowers. This new education produced a nationalistic robot-like people, obedient imitators, without the spirit of independence. It taught the youth of humanity to imitate the ideas and methods of the sages, which is impossible even for adults.

That's why, since the arrival of the seductive modern civilization, people immediately became slaves, not only materially but also spiritually. From this comes the necessity of discovering a new method of physiological and biological education.

At seventeen, I was struck with tuberculosis, and my condition was so serious that I was abandoned by modern medicine. I saved myself at the gates of death by the macrobiotic method. I would like to communicate to everyone the joy I feel in spreading this method to the entire world. This has been a self-education, as well as an education of the public.

Traditional Far Eastern medicine, originating five thousand years ago, was not a symptomatic medicine, but a fundamental method of cure that was based on understanding natural causes. This is why it was also a method of health, longevity, and happiness. It was not concerned with the disappearance of symptoms, but it was an educative medicine, which had as its end the development of man's judgment.

The primordial problem for man is the establishment of health. This is why we must give the greatest emphasis to education in health and hygiene. All living creatures except for man know how to control their own health. Modern medicine attaches all importance to the disappearance of symptoms. It does not search for the cause, and never tries to build up the source of vitality. Consequently, it has become a simple, specialized technique; it has fallen into mere formality, and its educative spirit has completely disappeared. That is why modern medicine vegetates in an impasse, in spite of formidable technical progress.

In the Far East, ancient education was, before all else, a way of independence—the study of the self, physiologically and biologically—and its goal was to follow a free and peaceful way through establishment of health by oneself, for oneself, and under one's control. The Far Easterners made a single way of medicine and education.

Thanks to the death of three of my nearest family members by the time I was eighteen years old, I vowed to discover the true cause of this absurd unhappiness, and by chance I found it. However, when I began to spread this practical method of life, I immediately encountered the second great problem of my life: the will.

If one lives correctly according to macrobiotic principles, all will go well and world peace can be rapidly realized. But the difficulty is that most people, especially the sick, don't have the will to hold to such a simple macrobiotic life. They lack will to such an extent that they prefer to submit to sickness and poverty, and are driven to crime. It is therefore necessary that a spiritual education, the education of the will, precede the reconstruction of society. Even after this revolution is made, if one neglects the education of the will, one will add to the production of salaried conformists who are slaves to their machines, robot-like observers who live blindly. Thus, in place of the creative spirit, the spirit of imitation is substituted, because those who create themselves and their own destiny are very small in number.

The fundamental basis of education is: 1. the self-control of health, and 2. the establishment of will. The first condition is resolved by applying the macrobiotic method. But by what educative method can one fortify the will? This second condition is the great problem. What is the great secret? What is will?

Education of the Will

In all times, great men—the free men, the sages—have proclaimed the importance of the will. No one denies it; everyone agrees that this is so. Nevertheless, most of humanity fails to use the will in everyday life, and life ends tragically for man after having known only "the glory of the bindweed" (a brief, ephemeral existence).

What are the reasons for this? What is the will? Are there many kinds or levels of will? Are there other conditions than the will alone for changing the destiny of man? Science keeps an absolute silence on these questions. This is normal. In the concept, or rather techniques, of modern scientific studies, the end of research is relative, limited, ephemeral, and physical. In other words, the focus is on the material world.

According to the thinking of the ancient Far East, which researched principally the infinite, absolute, eternal, constant, spiritual world, will has the following aspects:

- Will is a progressive form of judgment.
- There are seven stages of judgment, and therefore seven stages of will:

  1. Mechanical or blind
  2. Sensorial
  3. Sentimental or emotional
  4. Intellectual
  5. Social
  6. Ideological
  7. Supreme

- The seven stages or steps reflect the natural development of life. For example, in a plant the development is from seed to sprout to stalk to branches to leaves to flowers to fruits. Judgment or will is vitality itself. However, the first six steps have value only in the relative, limited world. Only the seventh is valid in the absolute world, as well as the relative world.

  Vitality, or the principle of development in nature, and the principle of the universe are the same. Vitality increases by the mutual sympathy of the two opposing elements, yin and yang: darkness and light, humidity and dryness, dilation and compression, centrifugal force and centripetal force, etc.

- The greatest mission of education is to make known the will, or "infinite expansion." When it is strong, it creates the man who has absolute health, who can try without trying, convince without speaking, order the mountain to enter the sea, conquer without fighting, govern the strong with gentleness, transmute the impossible into the possible, and accept difficulties with joy.

Since the will develops naturally and freely through seven stages, an artificial and exterior education is useless. Even though animals do not go to school, they develop in a perfect and sane way. They lead a free life, without sickness, without worries, without poverty, without scandalous pleasures. Instead of continuing the present system of education, it would be wise to discover a method of helping everyone to raise their judgment and change their thinking to one of deep appreciation and gratitude for their bosses, friends, and enemies. With this attitude it doesn't matter what we do—we are happy anytime, anywhere, without the crimes and wars that men are practicing now.

A small seed, which has neither force nor arms, accepts conditions of darkness, pressure, cold, and dampness. Instead of complaining or blaming others, it uses these conditions as sources of energy. It is trampled on and eaten by insects and worms, but with each difficulty it fortifies itself and develops more and more. Thus, man can lead a free life and be at peace with himself if he accepts it as a grain does; but, on the other hand, if he looks for artificial ease, comfort, pleasure, assistance, wealth, and security, or if he has an Epicurian conception of life—in the current degraded sense of the word—he will weaken his natural vitality.

It is therefore important for education to give the opportunity to know the natural origin of health—to teach the way to achieve health in every sense of the word. This way consists of using the correct foods, and combining, cooking, and eating them properly. As a consequence, one can discover and master by himself all the fundamental knowledge necessary to the social life of man, since judgment follows the process of its natural development. Those who, unhappily, have not received this education are the victims of natural selection, and will know only the suffering and difficulty of the world, the darkness of the seed and sprout. In time, many will fall in discouragement and become more and more unhappy, and manifest this unhappiness as criminals, slaves, and patients. The unhappy, the slaves, are the heavy burden of civi-

Ohsawa-Style Education

When I studied with George Ohsawa at his Maison Ignoramus school, we were free to go to bed at any time but had to wake up at 5:00 A.M. sharp. Sensei Ohsawa used to go to bed at 9:00 or 10:00 P.M. each night and woke at 1:00 or 2:00 in the morning. I remember often saying "good night" to him on my way to bed and receiving a good morning salutation from him because he had just woken up for the day.

The girl students were boarded at the house where Mr. and Mrs. Ohsawa were living. Some girls worked in the kitchen and the rest went out on sales trips for his weekly World Government *magazine. This was a part of his education to teach them how to behave in a gentle and agreeable way. All sales girls learned how to behave by selling in the street to strangers because they would sell more papers if they behaved better and more gently.*

We boys lived in a separate prefabricated house. It was a two-story building and the beds were like the beds of sleeping trains. We called them "silk worm beds." Our jobs were cleaning the house inside and outside, and editing the magazine. As long as people did some work in this school, ate the school meals, and gave answers to Ohsawa's daily questions, they were allowed to stay at the school. Ohsawa gave comment on students' answers to his questions at 8:00 every morning. It was not a usual school class but could be called "Ohsawa-style education."

His education was to teach humbleness, not arrogance; wisdom, not knowledge; self-reflection rather than blaming of others; and acceptance of another's faults while taking responsibility for one's own faults. Through question-and-answer sessions, students learned how to think for themselves, what their shortcomings were, and how to improve them. We learned much more than the knowledge taught at the University; we learned about life and ourselves.

Alcan Yamaguchi
Former owner of the first macrobiotic restaurant
in the United States

lized society, and they can become the cause of war. The responsibility for the existence of unhappiness belongs to the low judgment of parents and educators. However, these difficulties and sufferings are the indispensable touchstone for those who have supreme judging ability, since only these social evils can transmute discouragement into will.

During the many years that I have devoted to macrobiotic philosophy, I have spent more than twenty of them observing the educational programs of diverse Western countries. It is evident that their education is founded on the scientific knowledge which has built their civilization. For the most part, the teachings are techniques intended to aid adaptation to life. This means that it is a materialistic education, adapted to the physical world.

There exists no one single school, no one single university, dedicated to bringing forth and developing natural spontaneity, creative faculty, love—or in one word: instinct. However, the instinct of animals is a wonder to behold. Man has the same instinct. Were it not dulled and if we would learn to utilize it, what an infinite and outbursting joyfulness life would then bring us. For many centuries instinct has been too much neglected. We have been too preoccupied with the knowledge and progress of material civilization for our comfort and convenience. We have despised our instinct.

There are two categories of education: The first one develops, or rather reveals, more and more the innate supreme faculty of our perception, memory, comprehension, and judgment until it becomes a clearsightedness that gazes on the Order of the Universe. This contemplation operates through all finite, transient, and, in reality, illusory phenomena. It is love that embraces all things without any distinction, including the joyfulness that eternally and infinitely springs from it; that is to say, faith. The second category of education is really indoctrination. It teaches professional techniques and makes imitators and conformists, but veils or suppresses completely the inborn quality of the instinct or supreme judging ability. It is always those who have been educated in the second category who commit all kinds of felonies such as exploitation of the poor, wars, atom-bombing, etc.

The research of metaphysics, spirituality, will, supreme judgment, happiness, justice, peace, liberty, and infinite life was the specialty of thinkers or sages of the Far East for five thousand years. It is there that the five great religions of man were born, but these religions have since become excessively antiquated mummies.

Let us lay all this aside completely and start a new edition of the world, one that is neither physical nor metaphysical, but physical and metaphysical at the same time. It must provide the simplest and most practical method, which may be understood by all immediately and which is applicable in the daily life of all races. It is a new practical, physiological, and biological education. Its unique instrument is practical dialectics: an amusing algebra that resolves any difficult problem by employing yin and yang as the unknowns. Even children can understand it in an hour.

Education for a Peaceful World

Because of the gift of thought, the manner of man's reply to nature's offerings takes two antagonistic forms. One is harmonious adaptation; the other is the conquest of nature.

The first begins with innocent surprise, and, passing through the mysterious, ends with the discovery of the Order of the Universe. It leads finally to the world of peace, infinite gratitude, and universal identification. The second begins with fear rather than surprise and takes the path of destruction, killing, and conquest by violence, all by way of hate.

But it is the time of a new beginning when all must be remade. The history of humanity is now at the first line of the first page of the second volume.

Let us re-establish the world with our own hands. At first, re-education must be the way. This education establishes health first of all by its physiological and biological method. This is the setting in which the will appears: "a healthy spirit in a healthy body."

The education that will produce a new world, a free and peaceful world, begins with the creation of the healthy man. "You are what you eat," said Anthelme Brillat-Savarin. From my study of traditional Far Eastern medicine, and my many years of teaching it, I am more and more deeply and entirely convinced of the truth of these words, and I have arrived at this conclusion: If the nourishment is just, then the man is just.

I know of nothing more important for a human life and for society than the nourishment of the mother during the human embryonic period. It is the time of the fundamental construction of man's life. It is the period when the three-billion-year process of evolution is condensed into approximately two hundred eighty days. I see nothing that has a greater influence on human life than this nourishment during the embryonic period.

The physiological and biological education of childhood and youth is of the greatest importance after the embryonic period. If one gives macrobiotic nourishment from this age, one will make boys and girls who fulfill the seven conditions of health. Moreover, whoever fulfills these conditions realizes, by himself and for himself, a happy life. He becomes an independent man, who studies by himself. And a woman like this will be able to establish a happy family. She will devote herself to the construction of a happy and healthy society and country.

If you are willing to create a center that would contribute toward improving society, establish a little school and gather there a dozen children or students who have been condemned as inferior to their contemporaries. Teach them the Unifying Principle by day and by night, in theory and in everyday life, for six years. Then you will have given free men to society.

In the Far Eastern countries, the educational ideal is Zen, which is nothing more than a man provided with the Unifying Principle, supreme judging ability, and an understanding of the Order of the Universe. And education is synonymous with free life. In such a school, needless to say, there exist no lessons to commit to memory and no examination from memory; but there is living experience with a teacher who must be free, healthy, and of sound judgment.

You can well imagine that health derived from such an education would be soundly based, that a family built by those who enjoy such health would be happy indeed, that a society composed of such families would be strong, and that world peace can only be established by such societies working in unison.

In conclusion, I ask you to pose the following question to yourself: "What kind of an adult do I want my child to become—a doctor, a lawyer, a politician, a rich man, or the most happy, healthy, free human being?" Your answer will determine the direction that his education will take.

The education of the individual—the most important task that anyone can undertake—does not wait for the first day of preschool nursery or kindergarten to begin. It starts in the home long before that, for we influence our children from the very instant of conception.

Children are imitators. If their parents are interested only in material things like money and possessions, they will follow suit. They have no choice since during their formative years they are constantly in contact with the example that the parent sets.

If, however, you have educated yourself to understand that the true goal for man is an infinite one—the attainment of eternal happiness, supreme health, absolute justice, complete freedom— then your child's future is assured. Life with a happy, healthy, just parent is the most complete education of all.

How to "Eat" Books

As man nourishes with foods, he should carefully develop his spirit. All great or happy people have absorbed much more food of the spirit than physical foods. Books are of this invisible nourishment. As one can find foods of various qualities, from the best to the worst, likewise there exist all sorts of spiritual nourishment.

In general, food stores and restaurants are looking for business in offering us nourishment or meals, but they often neglect our health and happiness. As for the nourishment of the spirit, the goal of the bookstores is to sell to the maximum while awakening in the reader an agreeable sensation, his curiosity and his appetite, without taking into account his conception of life. Often what one calls a best seller disappears in two or three years because it is the modern technique of publishing that produced it. Therefore, if you have the intention of reading a good book, you should buy what was published at least twenty years ago. Books at least two hundred years old that one appreciates are certainly good. The book whose value has been recognized for two thousand years is the true best seller.

The Japanese have eaten rice for thousands of years. The Westerners have nourished themselves with wheat for a long time. These whole grains are, moreover, very cheap and have a good taste. Salt has been known for fifty thousand years as a necessary element of our nourishment. Curiously, the more the nourishment is "classic" the less expensive it is, and the most precious nourishment is nearly free. In that which concerns books, it is the same. The greatest and most precious book is nature. One cannot read it from A to Z even during an entire lifetime. To "masticate" this "book," one must absolutely possess special teeth called the Unifying Principle; otherwise, one cannot digest it.

One cannot apply the principle of *Shin-do-fu-ji* ("man is a product of his surroundings") to the nourishment of the spirit. Although the body (*shin*) and the surroundings (*do*) make one, the spirit cannot be identified since the body and its surroundings are finite while the spirit is infinite. The spirit knows not the limit of season, place, country, or weather. If one applies the principle of *Shin-do-fu-ji* to reading, one should read the "books of the season," and everyone should read equally the same books. It is truly funny. The best book in regard to the nourishment of the spirit is one that can sell itself in any country and any epoch. Briefly, there exists a great inequality between the order of the physical world and that of the world of the spirit.

But the Unifying Principle of yin and yang breaks down physical-world thoughts into their constituents and transforms them into proper nourishment of the spirit. In this case, the Unifying Principle plays the role of an enzyme, which acts as a catalyst. He who, as a cultivated macrobiotic student, desires to read all the books I recommend further on must first of all respect the function of the Unifying Principle. He who would possess the beautiful teeth of the Unifying Principle is never intoxicated, even by a poisonous book. Obviously, he must chew it well. Chewing transforms even toxins into nutritive substances.

What are excellent books? It is a matter of one's choice. I have recommended up until now more than three thousand books to my disciples in my monthly magazines. Since my youth, I have been in the habit of reading one book a day. I have spent much money on the nourishment of the spirit instead of wasting it at restaurants.

Recently, I read a book by Morton J. Adler called *How to Read a Book*. It defined the goal of reading as this: "Development of judgment to perfect oneself." In other words, that means, to my sense, how to search for infinite freedom and eternal happiness.

What is an excellent book? Adler replies, "The excellent book is simple and clear. Everyone understands it easily." This is a good definition. In our age, the best seller is successful for only one or two years. Mark Twain has defined an excellent book as follows: "Everyone knows about it, but no one reads it."

"When one has finished reading a book," writes Adler, "one is tired." That is not completely true. I can read any quantity of books without getting tired. I always find everything interesting. Reading is a work of the spirit and since the spirit is infinite and free, one never grows tired while reading. The body tires; the body is finite. But one does not read with the body, just as one does not cultivate the field with the spirit.

The macrobiotic reader, as a cultivated cosmopolitan personality, should at least have read the following books, which are all completely fundamental. They are listed in more or less chronological order. Moreover, these books represent only a part of those that I have already recommended. In any case, don't forget that a great number of excellent books await you.

1. *The Sacred Books of Buddhism*

2. *I-Ching*

3. Confucius: *The Analects*

4. Meng-tsu: *Mencius*

5. Lao-tsu: *The Tao-te-Ching*

6. Chuang-tsu: *Chuang-tsu*

7. Sen-Ma-Tsien: *Historical Memories*

8. Homer: *The Iliad; The Odyssey*

9. *The Bible (Old Testament)*

10. Aeschylus: *Prometheus Bound; Agamemnon*

11. Sophocles: *Oedipus the King; Antigone; Electra; Women of Trachis*

12. Euripedes: *The Medea; Electra; Hyppolytes; Bacchants*

13. Thucydides: *The History of the Peloponnesian War*

14. Hippocrates: *The Medical Works*

15. Aristophanes: *Lysistrata; The Birds; The Frogs*

16. Plato: *Crito; Phaedo; Phaedrus; Apology; The Republic; The Laws*

17. Aristotle: *Rhetoric; Politics; The Nicomachean Ethics; Poetics.*

18. Euclid: *The Elements of Euclid*

19. Cicero: *Philippics; Against Catiline; Against Verres*

20. Lucretius: *On the Nature of Things*

21. Virgil: *The Aeneid*

22. Horace: *Odes; Epodes; Poetic Art*

23. Ovid: *Metamorphoses; The Art of Love*

24. Plutarch: *Parallel Lives*

25. Cornelius Tacitus: *Germania; Annals*

26. Epictetus: *Discourses, Manual, and Fragments*

27. Lucian: *Dialogues of Death; Manner of Writing History*

28. Marcus Aurelius: *Thoughts*

29. *The Bible (New Testament)*

30. Saint Augustine: *The Confessions; On Grace; The City of God; Against the Pagans*

31. Mohammed: *The Koran*

32. *Nibelungenlied*

33. *The Song of Roland*

34. Saint Thomas Aquinas: *Summa Contra Gentiles; Summa Theologica*

35. Dante: *The Divine Comedy; The New Life*

36. Geoffrey Chaucer: *The Canterbury Tales*

37. Thomas à Kempis: *The Imitation of Christ*

38. Leonardo da Vinci: *The Literary Works of Leonardo da Vinci; Notebooks*

39. *Kojiki (Records of Ancient Matters)*

40. Lady Murasaki: *The Tale of Genji*

41. Niccolò Machiavelli: *The Prince*

42. Desiderius Erasmus: *The Praise of Folly*

43. Sir Thomas More: *Utopia*

44. Martin Luther: *Works*

45. John Calvin: *Institutes of the Christian Religion*

46. François Rabelais: *Gargantuas and Pantagruel*

47. Michel de Montaigne: *Essays*

48. Edmund Spenser: *The Faerie Queen*

49. Miguel de Cervantes: *The History of Don Quixote de la Mancha*

50. Sir Francis Bacon: *The Advancement of Learning; Indications Concerning the Interpretation of Nature*

51. William Shakespeare: *Hamlet; Othello; Macbeth; King Lear; The Merchant of Venice; Henry V; Richard II; Richard III; Henry VIII*

52. Galileo Galilei: *Dialogue on the Great World Systems*

53. William Harvey: *On the Circulation of the Blood*

54. Hugo Grotius: *The Rights of War and Peace*

55. Thomas Hobbes: *Leviathan*

56. René Descartes: *Discourse on Method; Meditations on the First Philosophy; Principles of Philosophy*

57. Pierre Corneille: *El Cid; Cinna; Horace*

58. John Milton: *Paradise Lost*

59. Molière: *The School for Wives; Don Juan; Tartuffe; The Misanthrope; The Doctor in Spite of Himself; The Imaginary Invalid; The Fourberies of Scapin; Amphitryon*

60. Baruch Spinoza: *Ethics; Political Treatice*

61. John Locke: *An Essay Concerning Human Understanding*

62. John Baptiste Racine: *Phèdre; Andromaque; Athalie*

63. Sir Issac Newton: *Mathematical Principles of Natural Philosophy*

64. Gottfried Wilhelm von Leibniz: *New Essays Concerning Human Understanding; Théodicés; Monadology*

65. Blaisse Pascal: *Pensées; The Provincial Letters*

66. Daniel Defoe: *Robinson Crusoe*

67. Jonathan Swift: *Gulliver's Travels; A Tale of a Tub*

68. Baron Charles de Montesquieu: *The Spirit of the Laws; Persian Letters*

69. François-Marie Arouet de Voltaire: *Zadig; Candide; Philosophical Letters*

70. Henry Fielding: *Tom Jones*

71. David Hume: *An Inquiry Concerning Human Understanding*

72. Jean Jacques Rousseau: *The Social Contract; Émile; Confessions*

73. Laurence Sterne: *The Life and Opinions of Tristam Shandy*

74. Adam Smith: *The Wealth of Nations*

75. Immanuel Kant: *Critique of Pure Reason; Critique of Practical Reason; Critique of Judgment; Fundamental Principles of the Metaphysics of Morals*

76. Edward Gibbon: *The Decline and Fall of the Roman Empire*

77. Marie Henri Beyle Stendhal: *The Red and the Black; The Charterhouse of Parma*

78. Johann Wolfgang von Goethe: *Faust; The Sorrows of Young Wether; Wilhelm Meister's Apprenticeship; Poetry and Truth*

79. David Ricardo: *The Principles of Political Economy and Taxation*

80. Thomas Robert Malthus: *Essay on the Principle of Population*

81. Georg Wilhelm Friedrich Hegel: *Phenomenology of the Mind; Science of Logic; The Philosophy of Right; Reason in History*

82. Auguste Comte: *System of Positive Polity*

83. Honoré de Balzac: *Father Goriot; Cousin Pons; Eugénie Grandet; Cousin Bette; Cesar Birotteau; The Research of the Absolute*

84. John Stuart Mill: *A System of Logic; Principles of Political Economy; On Liberty*

85. Charles Darwin: *The Origin of Species by Means of Natural Selection*

86. William Makepeace Thackeray: *Vanity Fair; The History of Henry Esmond*

87. Charles Dickens: *Oliver Twist; Pickwick Papers; David Copperfield; Christmas Tales*

88. Claude Bernard: *Introduction of the Experimental Medicine*

89. Karl Marx: *Communist Manifesto* (with Friedrich Engels); *Das Kapital*

90. Søren Kierkegaard: *The Concept of Dread; Sickness Unto Death*

91. Fedor Dostoevsky: *Crime and Punishment; The Idiot; The Brothers Karamazov*

92. Gustave Flaubert: *Madame Bovary; The Sentimental Education*

93. Hendrik Ibsen: *A Doll's House; Brand; Peer Gynt; The Wild Duck*

94. Leo Tolstoy: *War and Peace; Anna Karenina; Resurrection*

95. Friedrich Nietzsche: *Thus Spake Zarathustra; Beyond Good and Evil*

96. Emile Durckheim: *Suicide; The Elementary Forms of the Religious Life*

97. Richard Dedekind: *Continuity and Irrational Numbers*

98. William James: *Principles of Psychology; The Will to Believe; Pragmatism*

99. Ivan Petrovitch Pavlov: *Conditioned Reflexes*

100. Sigmund Freud: *The Psychopathology of Everyday Life; On Creativity and the Unconscious; An Outline of Psychoanalysis; A General Introduction to Psychoanalysis*

101. Jules Henri Poincaré: *Science and Method*

102. Lenin: *Materialism and Empirio-Criticism*

103. Marcel Proust: *Rembrance of Things Past*

104. George Bernard Shaw: *Pygmalion; St. Joan; Caesar and Cleopatra; Androcles and the Lion; Man and Superman*

105. Edmund Husserl: *Ideas: General Introduction to Pure Phenomenology*

106. Franz Boas: *The Mind of Primitive Man*

107. Henri Bergson: *Matter and Memory; Creative Evolution; The Two Sources of Morality and Religion*

108. Thomas Mann: *The Magic Mountain; Buddenbrooks; Dr. Faustus: The Life of the German Composer*

109. Albert Einstein: *Relativity: The Special and General Theory*

110. Leon Trotsky: *Literature and Revolution; The Russian Revolution*

111. James Joyce: *Ulysses; Portrait of the Artist as a Young Man; Finnegans Wake*

112. Kakuzo Okakura: *The Book of Tea*

113. Matsuo Bashō: *The Narrow Road to the Deep North*

114. Omar Khayyám: *Rubáiyát*

115. *The Thousand and One Nights*

116. Wu Ch'engen: *Hsi-yu chi* (partial English trans. *Monkey*)

117. *The Vedas*

118. *The Upanishads*

119. *The Cheda Sūtras*

120. Henry David Thoreau: *Walden*

121. Walt Whitman: *Leaves of Grass*

122. Oswald Spengler: *The Decline of the West*

123. S. Takata: *Correspondence and Words*

124. Mark Twain: *The Adventures of Tom Sawyer*

125. Jules Verne: *Twenty Thousand Leagues Under the Sea; Around the World in Eighty Days*

126. Lewis Carroll: *Alice in Wonderland*

127. Herman Melville: *Moby Dick*

128. Lin Yutang: *The Importance of Living*

129. Rabindranath Tagore: *East and West*

130. Eugen Herrigel: *Zen in the Art of Archery*

131. Shinran: *Tannishyo (The Treatise Which Deplores Heresy)*

132. Dōgen: *Shobogenzo Zuimonki (The Treasury of the Eye of the True Teaching)*

133. Nichiren: *Kaimokushō (The Opening of the Eyes)*

134. Hōnen: *Ichi Mai Kishomon (The Sermon on a Leaf)*

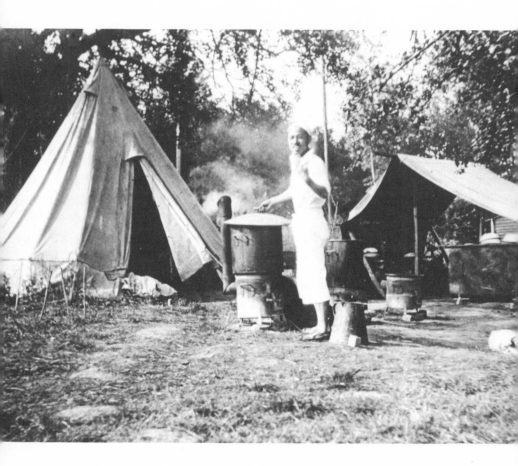

George Ohsawa preparing a meal at the International Peace Conference outside of Paris, August 19

5

THE UNIFYING PRINCIPLE OF YIN AND YANG

YIN-YANG CLASSIFICATION

In order that a science be useful, a logical, practical, fundamental, and universal classification is indispensable. The Unifying Principle is, in fact, a method of dialectical classification, practical and universal, attainable by all, embracing everything that exists in the universe and the universe itself. The traditional Far Eastern concept of life and universe is an absolute monism, although it appears at first glance to be a dualistic philosophy.

On one hand, the Unifying Principle is an analytical method, but on the other, it is a classification toward unification. The Unifying Principle divides all things into two antagonistic categories: yin and yang, according to the Chinese wise men. They are indeed two complementary forces indispensable to each other, like man to woman or day to night. They are the two fundamental and opposite factors that continually produce, destroy, and produce, repeatedly, all that exists in the universe.

Those phenomena that are more compounded with yang force than with yin are called yang, and vice-versa. Yin and yang exist in everything on an infinitely diversified scale. Satan existed even in Jesus and St. Francis, a fact that they both admitted. Daily we realize it within our own experience.

The Penniless Publisher

I first met this remarkable man (George Ohsawa) a few days after my arrival in Hiyoshi. I didn't have any money and spent the first couple of days in Tokyo looking for a job. My first evening at dinner, Ohsawa came to the table and distributed copies of Life, Time, Paris-Match, and other magazines and books from around the world. His dress and manner were very casual, not at all like a regular teacher. He wore a sports jacket and a cotton shirt open at the neck, and was puffing on a pipe. "Hello, what have you been doing today?" he would ask someone with a broad grin. "What do you think of this?" he would say to another, pointing to a headline or article in a magazine. His speech was very interesting, full of current affairs, skipping from events in Japan to the United States, Europe, and around the world. I realized I was in the presence of someone very unusual.

"Oh, you are the newcomer, aren't you?" he said with a penetrating stare through his black horn-rimmed glasses.

"Yes, I've just come from the country of Izumo," I replied.

"The letter you sent was a real waste of paper," he said sternly. "Next time, use only one sheet."

I had sent him a letter from Yokota, informing him that I would like to visit Hiyoshi and meet him. It had been written on several sheets of elegant stationery in a large, formal calligraphic hand with beautiful brush strokes. Later, I learned that he was a fanatic about paper. To a perpetually penniless writer and publisher like Ohsawa, paper and ink were like blood. They had often been scarce and expensive. Over the years, he acquired the habit of writing his manuscripts on the inside of old envelopes, on the back of grocery lists or laundry slips, and anything else that could be reused. He wrote in the smallest possible hand, often running to the edge of the sheet without leaving room for margins.

"What are you going to do?" he asked.

"I'm looking for work to survive," I replied.

He then asked the other students to evaluate my condition using the methods of traditional Oriental visual diagnosis they had learned in his lectures. The general conclusion was that my face was red from eating too much persimmon. He later dubbed me "the girl from the Izumo mountains with a face as red as a monkey's rump" because of my fondness for this fruit. I blushed in embarrassment but inside had to admit they had diagnosed correctly.

Aveline Kushi
Co-director of the Kushi Institute

From the physical point of view, that which contains more water (every other condition being equal) is yin; the reverse is true of yang.

In the chemical prospect, the compounds that are rich in hydrogen, carbon, lithium, arsenic, sodium, and magnesium are more yang than those that contain less of these elements and are rich in other elements, such as potassium, sulphur, phosphorus, oxygen, nitrogen, etc.

In short, yin and yang are always relative. There exists no one thing absolutely yin or absolutely yang in this world. "A" may be yin toward "B" but yang toward "C."

The characteristics of everything in the universe are due to the proportions and combinations of yin and yang. In other words, all phenomena and the character of all things are influenced by the two fundamental forces: the centripetal yang and the centrifugal yin. According to the Unifying Principle, anything may be classified as either yin or yang, then coordinated in accordance with respective proportions of the yin and yang constituents.

Centripetal yang produces the following phenomena: heat (thus, the activity of the molecular components); constriction; density; heaviness (thus, the tendency to go downward); flattened, low, horizontal forms. On the contrary, centrifugal yin produces:

cold (slackening of the components' movement); dilation; expansion; lightness (thus, the tendency to go upward); enlargement; tall, thin, vertical forms.

All that exists in this universe has a shape, color, and characteristic weight.

Shape: A,B,C,D are vertical forms; that is to say, they are ruled by centrifugal force.

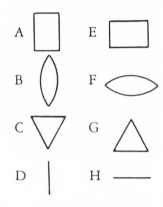

E,F,G,H are horizontal; e.g., they are dominated by the centripetal force.

Two by two, these figures have the same geometrical surface, but they are antagonistic: One is yin, the other yang. In particular, antagonisms between C and G and D and H are very accentuated.

In this shape, which is divided in half by a horizontal line, you see three times more centrifugal force ▼ than centripetal ▲ force. D and H superimposed make a cross; C and G, the Judaic star. They are sacred symbols, representing a unification of yin and yang.

Weight: Centripetal force governs that which is heavy and therefore yang. Centrifugal force dominates that which is lighter and therefore yin. The lighter in weight, the more yin.

Color: Our very first perception of this world is in color. Without color we can see nothing. To classify colors is very easy. The color that you feel is the warmest and the one that you feel is the coldest are the two yang and yin extremes respectively. All other degrees of warmth and cold lie between them. Everybody knows them. They are represented by red, orange, yellow, green, blue, indigo, and violet. It is the natural order of colors that one sees in the spectrum when natural light is refracted by a prism, or in the rainbow. This can be verified by thermometry. Generally speaking, yin foods are outwardly or internally bluish or violet in color; yang foods are red or yellow.

You can now discriminate between yin and yang in everything in the universe: by shape, by weight, and by color.

You can classify light and the radiations from wavelengths. The longer the waves, the more yang they are (red, infrared); the shorter the wavelength, the more yin (violet, ultraviolet).

All other biological, physiological, physical, and logical characteristics such as chemical composition, tropism, geographical location (and the bioecological one) of natural products, as well as their aptitude to adaptation, etc., may be classified yin and yang by means of the three fundamental characteristics (shape, weight, color), without the use of instruments or analytical methods. You can similarly classify disease, microbes, and all the factors that introduce illness.

Water: All other elements being equal, that which contains more water is more yin than that which is drier. Quantitatively, water is the most important compound in our body, but in excess it can reduce our vitality, since this means a dilution of blood (anemia). It lowers our body temperature and our cells become limited in sustenance. Our heart and kidneys become tired, for they are compelled to overwork.

One who holds more water has less centripetal (yang) force and more centrifugal (yin) force. Water is constantly evaporating since it is dominated by centrifugal (yin) force. Generally speaking, those who are very active drink much more water than those who are not. This is quite understandable, as they lose their body's water through activity, and are thirsty. Those who are not very active but drink a great deal of liquid become yin, chilly, more inactive, lazy, shy, and weak.

If you water a dry grain that generally contains only 13 percent water, it inflates, decomposes (yin), and the germ (yin) grows (yin) to become a plant. All these activities are yin (expansive). You are quieter when it rains, but you feel much more active and happy when the weather is fine (less humid), especially if you suffer from rheumatism. This means that rheumatism is a yin disease.

You can thus cure it by drinking less water and eliminating from your diet all that is rich in water. But if you are greedy for sugar or sugared sustenance, drinking less is not enough, for in our body sugar turns into water and carbon dioxide; both decrease the amount of yang elements in our blood and increase the proportion of potassium to sodium.

A great many vegetarian naturalists enjoy simple food, but what they like most is always sugar or something artificially sugared by industrial and commercial chemical sugar. Sugar is the unequaled number one murderer in the whole history of humanity. It is the most yin of all foods and the cause of numerous fatal diseases.

Chemical and industrial refined sugars differ from the natural variety, which contains all the minerals, proteins, oils, and vitamins we need to maintain our vitality. Refined sugar completely lacks these elements. Besides, it contains many chemical products that are very detrimental to health. Sugar is the greatest evil that modern industrial civilization has introduced in the countries of the Far East and Africa. It is much more murderous than opium and wars, particularly for those who eat rice as their principal food.

In the times of Jesus, Buddha, and Lao-tsu, people did not know this chemical and industrial poison. This is quite apparent, because they did not speak of it. But were they alive today, they would be the first to advise us against it.

Chemical Composition: The best potassium/sodium proportion is 5 to 1. All those foods with a ratio greater than 5 to 1 are yin, and those smaller than 5 to 1 are yang. For example: Egg is 1 to 1; whole brown rice is 5 to 1; potato is 512 to 1; orange is 570 to 1; banana is 850 to 1. (These ratios can vary quite significantly according to the use of fertilizers and other chemicals.) If yin foods are eaten exclusively, death will occur in weeks or months, depending on the strength of one's constitution.

How can one define potassium as yin and sodium as yang? I define them quantitatively and qualitatively by the agricultural, chemical, physical, physiological, and especially spectroscopical experimental method. Sodium may be considered as being a representative or symbol of the yang elements, and potassium of the yin elements. The potassium/sodium function is very practical since sodium and potassium are found in almost all chemical compositions of living things. Thus, they are two important indicators of the two groups of elements, yin and yang. Calcium and magnesium are two other indicators.

The complementary antagonism between sodium and potassium that plays so important a part in our physical as well as spiritual life was discovered by a Japanese doctor, Sagen Ishizuka, in the late 1900s. At that time he had already cured some hundreds of thousands of people . . . people who had been condemned and abandoned as incurable. He was so famous that letters addressed only to *Dr. Anti-doctor, Tokyo*, would reach him. When he died, his funeral escort was over two miles long.

At present, I am practically his only successor. His discovery was a new biochemical interpretation of the Unifying Principle, which dates back five thousand years. I developed it one step further, from the medical biochemical theory to the Unifying Principle of infinite freedom, eternal happiness, and absolute justice through universal logic, for everyone. World peace can be established only by adopting this Unifying Principle, which maintained peace and freedom for Far Eastern peoples for so many thousands of years, if it is translated and taught by a scientific, educational world institution such as UNESCO, WHO, or the UN.

As a matter of fact, the complementary antagonism between sodium and potassium is the key that reveals life's great secrets by the system of our sympathetic nerves, generator of all our physiological and psychological activities.

But there are still many other chemical elements and physical factors that play a more or less important part in this complementary antagonism, as I have already shown by some examples. Accordingly, this potassium/sodium antagonism is not to be exaggeratedly insisted upon, nor is the importance of sodium and potassium to be overemphasized, as by some Western physiologists. For, indeed, the potassium/sodium ratio can differ considerably among various specimens of the same plant. Even in a single carrot, for instance, it is different in the upper part as compared to the lower.

Geographical Point of View: All things that live in cold regions, all that are produced and grow more easily in the coldest countries, are yang compared with those which adapt themselves better in warm climates. If there is more diarrhea in hot than in cold countries, it stems from the fact that there are many more yin foods growing in the warmer than in the colder countries; diarrhea (i.e., cholera) is caused by an extraordinary dilation of the intestines (dilation and expansion are always yin), by yin factors (physical, chemical, physiological, biological, microbiological, or sociological), of which the strongest is always in food. The basic cause of diarrhea being so simple, its cure is extremely easy.

People who live in the Nordic and cold countries are always physiologically stronger than those who live in the southern ones (in the northern hemisphere), since they eat more yang foods, which are more easily produced in a yin (cold) climate than a yang (hot) climate. Moreover, yin beings do not adapt themselves easily to a yin climate, as is pointed out in the third of the Twelve Theorems of the Unifying Principle (see page 128). This explains why the five Big Walls (the *Maginot Line* included) were erected by the southern peoples to protect themselves from the more yang peoples coming from the north.

Elephants adapt themselves better in a warm and watery country. This means they are very yin. The fact that there were mammoths in Siberia thousands of years ago indicates this country then had a more temperate climate.

Taste: We can distinguish yin from yang by taste as well as by smell. The gradations from yin to yang are: hot or pungent (like the pimento which gives a sensation of warmth by dilating our capillaries and increasing the blood flow); sour; sweet; salty; bitter.

One must remember that these tastes are natural and not artificial or chemical. The sweetness of refined sugar is a hundred times greater than that of natural sweetness. If you want to locate chemical refined sugar on our qualitative scale of yin and yang, you will find it far out on the yin end.

Adaptability: Wild herbivorous animals must search constantly for plant-sources of energy. Local and seasonal variations as well as other biological and bioecological circumstances sometimes drastically limit food supply. But being blessed with adaptive functions that develop in inverse proportion to the poverty of their supply, they are able to build proteins necessary to their species. This great productive capacity, variable and elastic, fluctuates according to nitrogen supply and overall living conditions. In particular, more protein is produced in winter when plant food frequently diminishes, whereas in summer, generally a time of abundance, production is curtailed.

Yin produces yang and yang produces yin. This is a fundamental law of life, which is completely ignored by modern biology and physiology.

You can now understand why wild animals grow fatter in a cold climate that is apparently hostile and unfavorable. The dialectical adaptability of all wild or natural animals permits production of more protein during winter. Another way of putting it is to say that cold (yin) stimulates adaptability and productivity (yang).

Man's discovery of fire and salt marked the beginning of civilization. Fire and salt, two important factors of yangization, enabled man to obtain at will warmth and energy from the outside. As a result, he lost a measure of resistance to cold, eventually being forced to wear clothes. Naturally, the more clothes he wore, the more susceptible to cold he became. This is dialectical logic in dynamic action: the greater the utility, the greater the inutility.

Fire and salt, while decreasing man's yang adaptive abilities, also increased the yin side of his nature, resulting in greater sensitivity, sentimentality, and exclusiveness. Growing gradually less capable of producing his own proteins, man turned to more frequent meat-eating in an effort to obtain them. But the more animal proteins he consumes, the more dependent he becomes on lower species. Growing lazier and lazier (in other words, more and more "civilized"), he no longer hunts or even raises cattle for himself.

Foods: Diet is the most important factor in the phenomena of life and physiology and especially in the womb of the mother. Its importance is inestimable. In the development of the fetus we clearly see the influence of yin and yang, expansion and contraction. The proportions of these two factors in food determine the shape of all creation.

Salt, for example, is very yang. It toughens and brings things together. It can be used anywhere, at any time. If one cooks beans with a little salt, it is difficult to soften them. If one adds some salt before cooking potatoes, they do not lose their shape.

Many elements are antagonistic to the forces of salt—for example, water, sugar, potassium, sulphur, oxygen, and nitrogen. If potatoes are cooked with much water or some sugar, they become a shapeless mass.

Today, radishes, sweet potatoes, rice, and wheat are larger (more swollen) than in former years because they are cultivated with chemical fertilizers (sulfur, nitrogen, phosphorus)—all antagonistic to salt. Yet, without the elements that soften, disjoin, and separate them, vegetables and man become small, rigid, and dwarflike.

Let us perform a bit of discrimination: Which are the most yin among fruits and vegetables? If you wish to strengthen your practical discrimination, investigate and then jot down your answers on a sheet of paper.

Generally speaking, the most yin are eggplant, figs, red raisins, red cabbage (violet, indeed), the germ of the potato, oranges (particularly if violet inside), sugar (sugar cane), etc. All are outwardly or internally bluish or violet in color. All are very rich in potassium and vitamin C; all are very yin. Yang foods are red or yellow: meat and all the products from hemoglobin, fish, eggs, vitamin D, etc. They are rich in sodium in comparison to potassium.

In order to confirm this, eat a bit more of these yin foods than usual every day for a week and you will notice that you will become more yin in proportion to the extra amounts of yin you ate. Of two individuals under identical dietetic conditions, he who constantly eats yin foods will become more chilly and have less resistance to cold, compared with the one who does not eat them.

If you gave these foods to your child every day, you would see him become more and more yin (inactive, chilly, silent) and if he were tubercular (a yin illness), he would soon die.

If you gave these foods to a pregnant woman every day for some weeks (or even days), her delivery would be difficult and untimely;

the baby could even be stillborn. The sterile woman and those who are prone to premature delivery generally have a great liking for these foods. Children whose eyes are too far apart, or are myopic or lame, as well as those who have bad memory and do not like to learn, or are physically weak, are victims of this kind of diet.

The depopulation of a country or territory producing many fruits (rich in potassium and vitamin C) is consequently quite natural.

Food gives us life and vitality, but it can kill us very easily if we absorb it in bad proportions and if it is badly prepared. I could give you a murderous dietetic prescription with which you could kill yourself in a few days, eating very delicious ordinary foods. With these foods you could kill a very strong and healthy person in the space of some days or weeks, without ever being suspected, and without taking the chance of missing, as one might with a pistol.

Chemical Elements: The group of chemical elements with yang characteristics is composed of hydrogen (H), carbon (C), lithium (Li), sodium (Na), magnesium (Mg), and arsenic (As). At the forefront of the yin group stands oxygen (O); then come nitrogen (N), potassium (K), phosphorus (P), and the vast majority of all other chemical elements.

Biologists know that life on earth cannot exist without sodium or potassium. All living beings contain both. The proportion, however, varies with the characteristics of each species, its birth, and its way of living. Although some few species with very simple structures do live without these elements, such species still require a combination of two main elements (for instance, hydrogen and oxygen or carbon and oxygen) in a relationship of yin and yang opposition.

Balance: Our health and vitality depend on the simultaneous introduction of yin foods and yang foods in proportions that will lead to the establishment of a normal human balance.

If yin becomes absolutely dominant in the constitution of a living being, such a living being will disappear. The same result follows absolute dominance of yang. Insuring a balanced proportion between yin and yang is of utmost importance. Bearing that in mind, we can assert that there is no poison in nature, only a lack of harmony, an improper balance between yin and yang (centri-fugality and centripetality).

An organism with a stable constitution will be able to absorb and neutralize any unbalanced product—up to a certain point. In fact, we can even extend this theory to its ultimate by saying that healthy organisms can absorb and neutralize any poison. The historic case of the monk Rasputin is an example of this capacity pushed to the extreme.

In their actions as well, men exhibit opposing tendencies that can also be classified as yin or yang. When faced with a problem such as, for example, a constitutional disease, some men react with fear. Gradually or quickly, depending on the individual, this fear (yin) evolves into hostility (yang), which is expressed in violent attacks aimed at total suppression of symptoms. The cause, generally ignored, soon finds other means of externalizing itself. Thus, a chain of summary acts of violence disturbs and deterio-rates the internal environment and, if unchecked, leads to death. The infernal prospect of nuclear war is a global equivalent of man's fear-inspired brutalization of himself.

Distinguishing Yin and Yang: Table 5.1 summarizes various phenomena as consequences of the two fundamental forces, yin and yang.

You have now understood how to distinguish yin from yang, but all methods may be imperfect; their synthesis being more or less intricate for beginners, I shall suggest another method, very practical and easy.

Biologically, all animals are only converted vegetables, hemo-globin being a mutation of chlorophyll. Our physical, psychological, and even spiritual condition depends upon the proportion and the preparation of our foods, as well as upon our way of eating. The yin-yang proportion must always be 5 to 1. But, during the prepara-tion of foods, physical (heat, pressure) and chemical (salt, water) factors change this rate by decomposing, evaporating, diluting, con-densing, and combining elements of the original composition of the food. It is thus difficult to strictly maintain the 5-to-1 ratio.

A very easy and practical method for everyone consists in daily examining your fecal matter and urine with respect to color, shape,

Table 5.1 Classifying Phenomena as Yin or Yang
Physical

	Yin	Yang
Tendency	expansive	contractive
Position	outward	inward
Structure	space	time
Direction	ascent (up)	descent (down)
Color	purple (violet)	red
Temperature	cold	hot
Weight	light	heavy
Factor	water	fire
Atomic	electron	proton
Element	potassium (K)—the representative yin element. All elements in the periodic table (O, P, Ca, N, etc.) are yin excepting the few listed in the next column as yang.	sodium (Na)—the representative yang element. The yang elements in the periodic table are: H, As, C, Li, Na, Mg.

Biological and Physiological

	Yin	Yang
Biological	vegetable	animal
Agricultural	salad	cereal
Sex	female	→ male
Nervous System	sympathetic parasympathetic	
Birth	cold season	hot season
Movement	passive	active
Taste	sweet, sour, hot	salty, bitter
Vitamins	C	A, D

Bioecological

	Yin	Yang
Country of Origin	tropical	frigid
Season	growth in summer	growth in winter

and weight. If your urine is deep brown and transparent, if your evacuations are dark orange or brown and in substantially good shape, long and buoyant, and with a good smell, it is a sign that your diet of the previous day was chemically and physically in good proportion of yin and yang. If they are too bright, you have eaten too much yin. A yellow, transparent urine, giving sediments after about ten minutes, reveals a more or less severe illness, such as kidney disease, either because of an excess of calories or a lack of yang factors. If very diluted, transparent, and copious, it shows the probability of diabetes. He who must urinate more than four times a day (twenty-four hours) is already ill with tired kidneys, heart disease, etc. If you are constipated, or if you evacuate more than twice a day, you already have more or less serious troubles. If the stools are greenish and easily oxidized (blackening), there is a large excess of yin. He who is healthy needs little or no toilet paper, like all animals in nature.

In every case, the color of your evacuations must be deep orange or brown, agreeable to be seen, like an omelette (a bit overcooked), and have an agreeable scent, too. A bad smell indicates a bad working of the stomach and intestines.

Our physiological life and our activities depend completely upon our food, which should always be based on whole grains and vegetables. For man, they provide proper yin-yang balance, as opposed to animal products. Vegetable life and production depends on chlorophyll. If we eat the products of chlorophyll, they are transformed into hemoglobin and thus one partakes of cellular nutrition. We discard in orange or yellow products (bowel movements, urine) all that cannot be transformed into red blood. In other words, our physiological life is but a process that changes chlorophyllous products into red hemoglobinic blood. This process creates yang out of yin products.

The culinary preparation of food makes this physical and chemical transformation of vegetables into real human compounds easy, thanks to the yang factors (salt, fire, pressure, dehydration). This is why the utilization of fire and the discovery of salt were so important and significant. They made possible the best and the worst of human civilization, differentiating man from the animals. The unique system of yin and yang functions unceasingly in our digestive organs: carbohydrates (the most yang) are digested by saliva in the mouth (the most yin location); protein (more yin than carbohydrates but more yang than fats), by secretions produced by the stomach (more yang in location than the mouth);

and oils and fats (the most yin), in the intestines (the most yang in terms of location).

Our physiological life is a transmutation of yin colors to yang ones. Our health, happiness, and freedom depend on that transmutation. How simple it is. This is life. Here is one of life's great secrets. Its antithesis, death, is faulty diet, which produces the ridiculous and tragic moving pictures of the materialistic world, e.g., widespread illness and war. Having understood the basic cause, we need only to apply our knowledge.

In principle, life is quite simple. It is created, animated, decomposed, and reproduced by a dualistic, polarizable-monistic principle. But this dualism is not only one of sodium and potassium: there are yin and yang factors infinitely. We have to unify all of them and find out the monistic principle that creates all these dualisms. The antagonistic chemical and physical elements must be directed and balanced in a harmonious way toward health and happiness. The understanding of the Unifying Principle was born long ago in the Far East. Our task is to apply this knowledge to avert the catastrophic end of civilization through incurable sickness, atomic warfare, and planetary destruction.

Modern medicine exhibits no real concern for the causes of disease. It is totally ignorant of the cause of the common cold and, in fact, does not even search for it. Its prime concern is palliative treatment that will suppress a patient's symptoms. It is not even bothered by the fact that its search for a symptomatic remedy has proved fruitless.

Why, instead of looking for a fundamental, unifying, and permanent solution to the problems of disease, does official medicine prefer an endless series of symptomatic, palliative, and temporary solutions? My conclusion is that the source of this failure is man's own dualism or separatism, diversely manifested in the oppositions of spiritualism-materialism, selfishness-altruism, science-philosophy, God-man, body-soul, ad infinitum. And from what source does such dualism spring? From nothing less than a very real sclerosis, the death of brain cells.

The "precision instrument" of modern civilization—science— is blind; its faculties of judgment are still impaired. Without a practical technique, philosophy becomes useless, while at the same time a technique without a guiding principle is absurd and often dangerous. The best proof of this is the danger under which the whole of humanity lives today—nuclear annihilation.

It is curious to notice that many are pursuing their studies without even knowing that they are dualistic:

- Materialists, as well as spiritualists or idealists, who are convinced that there exist matter and spirit. They begin with the fundamental antagonism between materiality and spirituality. They want to exclude or abolish their opponents; they are exclusive. Thus, they are dualists, at least until they show how and by what mechanism all spiritual and ideal phenomena are produced. They must establish first of all their concept of world cosmology, which should explain what life and the universe are for everyone. Otherwise, their philosophy is nothing but a simple hypothesis or postulate.
- Pacifists, who are born out of the antagonism between peace and war.
- Physicians, who have busied themselves with "devil's bullets," which are fabrications that attempt to annihilate all the factors that cause humanity to suffer. They view symptoms and disease as bad; they do not understand them as alarms announcing disorder in the total organism; thus, they are dualists.
- All theologians who endeavor to distinguish man from God. They also are dualistic in viewing Satan against God.
- The psychosomatic or the Freudian schools, for example, which are new dualistic viewpoints in medicine and psychology.

Nearly all scientific and cultural researchers nowadays are, knowingly or not, dualistic. This is the reason why, instead of being solved, problems are more and more multiplied or ramified. All professionals, including politicians, educators, and all those who strive to destroy evil or to increase comfort, are dualists.

Descartes' dichotomy was the first step to monism. This first step has been much admired, but no one has ventured to go beyond the level of dichotomy. We must go a step further.

Dualism is exclusive and egocentric. Its weapons are destructive, analytical, and rough, whereas real monism is constructive, synthetical, and unifying. Life itself is always productive, unifying, and social, while the opposite is true of death.

Monism or the Unifying Principle is man's universal compass or direction-finder, pointing the way toward an awareness of eternal happiness, infinite freedom, and absolute justice.

SEVEN LOGICAL PRINCIPLES

Complementary antagonism is the definitive characteristic of this illusory and relative world. The relative world exists as an infinitesimal geometric point of incessant change within the one absolute and infinite world, which is beyond time-space and without limitation or restriction. This relative world is a theater of performances in which all the tiny and ephemeral parts are woven together in endless variations. The great universe itself, however, is one unified existence without beginning or end. The great universe is an ocean of absolute infinite expansion, while the relative world is a world of fleeting and transitory sense data, which is continually multiplying. The universe is infinite not only in time and expansive space, but also within the geometrical constitution of each of the individual elements or parts existing within that great expanse.

The drama of this relative world, however, is not without order. It is not mere chaos. There is a clear lineage of natural order that each and every person, primitive or modern, is living within and according to. For example: summer and winter; heat and cold; day and night; humidity and dryness; male and female; beginning and end; activity and passivity; ascending and descending; growth and diminution; blossoming and withering; centripetal and centrifugal force; constriction and dilation; construction and destruction; rest and movement; fast and slow—all of these opposing factors are in constant contrast and conflict. Taken together these opposites are but the two ends of a spectrum. Although opposing each other, they are also attracted to each other under the influence of a superior force; they keep crossing and exchanging their positions. These opposites are, in fact, the very reason why so-called evolution goes on within nature at an increasing rate of speed.

A Larger View

I met George Ohsawa in the summer of 1965. The occasion was "Camp Satori" held in the Feather River Country of California. Having done some reading on Zen Buddhism, I was embarrassed by the camp's name. Satori is a state achieved after many years of rigorous discipline—not after only ten days of good eating.

I enjoyed Mr. Ohsawa's blunt English and his profound sense of humor. While apologizing for his lack of English speaking skills, he communicated very well with short phrases, or often just a snort of a laugh.

The latter arose when we gave him our pitiful answers to his questions. His classes were perplexing to me. An honor roll student through high school and college, I had always been able to play the academic game quite easily. I would figure out what the teachers wanted and give it to them. But how could I give Mr. Ohsawa "correct" answers when I couldn't begin to figure out what he wanted. For the first time in my life, I felt stupid.

At the last lecture of the last day, Mr. Ohsawa was returning our written answers to some questions he had posed. He said he had been disillusioned by our lack of comprehension, but finally he could detect some growth. One question had been, "What is your revolutionary response to 'That which has a beginning has an end'?"

Ohsawa would read the answer he rated most highly. He would put an "x" on poor answers, one circle for adequate, and two circles for good. In this case, he had drawn three concentric circles, saying that this answer made the camp worthwhile to him. He asked whose it was and I raised my hand. "You?" he asked incredulously, remembering my earlier ignorant answers, "You are the author?" Then he asked to keep it.

When I had written my answer, I had at last managed to get beyond academic thinking. No longer seeking the rational, out of desperation, my mind expanded—I took a larger view. Here it is:

For the first time I see that the technological rise of the West can end in something other than disaster, whether big bang or ecological strangulation. If man began to violate the natural order, to attempt the domination of nature, he will stop doing so. My job must be to study this beginning to seek ways of transmuting the violation. A more difficult job I cannot imagine. It is almost like a leaf floating on a great river saying, "I shall reverse the flow."

George Ohsawa particularly liked the last sentence.

As we drove down the rice-growing valley towards home, we were very grateful for Ohsawa's teaching, and for the presence of his beautiful wife, Lima, who had so enjoyed seeing our baby daughter. We seemed very different people from the ones who had driven up the valley just ten days before. Perhaps the camp was not so badly named after all.

Mathew Davis
Artist

So that all people can understand the order that exists behind the seeming chaos of this world, I would like to present you with seven extremely fundamental and universal laws.

1. Whatever has a beginning has an end (the principle of inversion and the negation of the law of identity and contradiction in time). That which has a beginning is inevitably proceeding toward its opposite. Beginning and ending are always opposed to each other: birth-death; formation-decomposition; poverty-wealth; meeting-separating; having-losing, etc.

   In this way, all of these various functions are inverted forms of their opposite. All things in this relative world, at a greater or lesser pace, will eventually conform to this law.

   If there is anything that does not conform to this law, it belongs to the absolute, infinite world. Such a thing, however, is exceedingly rare. You must be extremely careful in order to detect the invisible and infinite thread that runs through and connects all things.

2. That which has a front has a back (the principle of *omote-ura*, front and back in Japanese, and the negation of the law of identity and contradiction in space). Front and back are opposites and they are also complementary. There is nothing in this world that has one without the other. The surface of a Gobelin tapestry and its reverse side are inseparable and yet opposed. A new weapon invites another superior weapon; profit is always accompanied by some aspect of loss. The streets of modern cities are filled with crime. Joy and suffering are twins.

3. No two things are identical (principle of difference and the negation of the law of identity). There are no two identical things in this world. Mountains, rivers, rocks, states and countries, the Earth and other planets, the sun and stars, people: all are unique.

4. The larger and greater the front, the larger and greater the back (the principle of balance and the negation of the law of the excluded middle).

   When one reaps great profits in some way, one inevitably receives great losses in another. Great progress is accompanied by great degeneration. One example is the striking contrast of modern civilization and nuclear warfare. The legal system and the police are always running a competitive marathon with crime. It is the same with modern medicine and disease.

5. Change (differentiation or movement), as well as stability (state of temporary equilibrium as two opposing forces exchange their energy and direction), are products of the two fundamental, universal, and dialectical forces of yin (centrifugality) and yang (centripetality) confronting each other (principle of dual origin and the negation of formal logic).

   The forces of yin and yang are interpreted as cold-hot; dark-light; acid-alkaline; dilation-constriction; ascent-descent; negative-positive; feminine-masculine, respectively. These are all antagonistic and at the same time complementary.

   Everything is in a state of constant, incessant change. All

is fluctuating, volatile, and ephemeral. All is engaged and in motion. Motion, differentiation, joining together, separation, creation, and decomposition are all nothing more than the various processes of change through which all things must inevitably pass. Mountains are waves that rise and fall within empty space and then subside and vanish into nothing. Change is everything. Balance or equilibrium is the point where two different directions meet and exchange their respective energies. All changes, as well as so-called balance or equilibrium, are produced and given life by the intersecting of opposites. The resulting scene is then projected onto the screen of the absolute or infinity.

6. The two conflicting forces of yin and yang are the right and left hands of the one, absolute, eternal infinity (principle of polarization and the foundation of the universal dialectic logic).

Since yin and yang are in reality complementary, all phenomena have a dialectical constitution made of these two opposing factors. All physical phenomena contain a central point that gathers all peripheral elements toward its center. Furthermore, all chemical elements are made up of two groups that continually contend with each other. For this reason, one uses the reactionary changes of opposing factors such as acid and alkaline and heat and cold alternatively for physical or chemical analysis and synthesis. Without antagonism there is also nothing complementary. Yin and yang are the two hands that create, sustain, and destroy, in order to produce anew, everything that exists in this relative world. Therefore, all things existing are inevitably relative, antagonistic, and, at the same time, complementary. Where there is no conflict, there is also no harmony. Where there is no contradiction, there is also no agreement. Therefore, every thesis is progressing towards antithesis in order to synthesize and create a new thesis.

I believe, at this point, it should be obvious that the above six principles, all of the relative world, completely destroy all the old laws or theories. These are, after all, of no use whatsoever in solving the disputes and quarrels of everyday and

family life, much less international conflicts, which require
an even larger perspective in order to be understood. Formal
logic is an extremely sensory and simple-minded invention.
The law of identity is demolished without a sound by the
principle of inversion, as is the law of the mean by the
principle of balance.

7. This great universe, the so-called world of oneness, is unchanging, limitless, constant, and omnipotent. It is infinity
   itself and produces, transforms, increases, destroys, and
   gives rebirth to all people and things both physical and spiritual (principle of polarizable monism).

     This oneness may be referred to as God, the all-knowing,
   all-powerful, and ever-present One; the ruler of the universe;
   that primal force that is uncreated and without beginning or
   end; the infinite, eternal, One.

     Principles one through six appeal to the five senses. They
   are a sketch of the order of the relative world. They are the
   most fundamental principles underlying the entire manifest
   world, from the earth we live on to the great expanse of the
   universe. In contrast to these, the seventh principle is a sketch
   of the parental source of yin and yang, the ultimate cause of
   the universe itself.

These principles are, first of all, dynamic; that is why they are
opposite to formal logic, which is static. They can be applied to any
domain, at any stage of life, and to all things existing in the relative
universe. Moreover, they can unify all antagonisms.

Formal logic is rigid; it is a simple snapshot of life in the
infinite universe, thus, infinitesimally analytical without intend-
ing or knowing; whereas universal logic is a living image of all life
and all things. Formal logic destroys continuity. The law of identity
and contradiction and the law of the excluded middle show us only
a static, finite image, an image imprisoned in the static world, determined from appearance, built on our senses or our instruments.

In reality, all things in this world change, ceaselessly, from one
extreme to the other. Nothing is stable or constant in this relative world.
Those who do not see this fact look for constants. And everything

they think to be constant is only an instantaneous "snapshot," an illusory, non-living, and infinitesimal part of the infinite and eternal universe. Analytical eyes are blind in the infinite universe.

Rather, it is these seven principles that do not change. Together, they constitute the Order of the Universe, and this order is the only eternal truth in our world. This is the foundation of all universal logic or theory. In fact, the only school of logic that is truly universal and eternal is that which is correctly established on this order. All things ideological or social, as well as physical, that are not based on this order will sooner or later be destroyed by their own inertia, fall into the chaos that they have invited, and finally perish altogether.

All scientific and cultural laws are based on the laws of physical nature, which, in turn, are based on the Order of the Universe. This order is the creator of all the various complex manifestations of this world and therefore seems on the surface to be extremely complex, while in actuality it is quite simple. If its essence is not understood, it will be impossible to establish world government or a world constitution. If we intuitively grasp this unique truth, the Order of the Universe, and make it a part of our own being, we will be able to manifest whatever we dream. "Seek first the kingdom of heaven and its justice and all else shall be added unto you." (Matthew 6:33.)

The kingdom of heaven of which Jesus spoke is none other than the absolute, eternal, infinite world spoken of in the seventh principle. The justice of this kingdom is none other than the eternally unchanging Order of the Universe that guides and leads all things to their intended perfection. If you once make this order into your own understanding, you will be able to resolve all conflicts and make all antagonisms complementary. Jesus and Lao-tsu were among those few great sages who discovered the universal order. Jesus called it "divine justice" and stated that "All words are from the mouth of God." The famous words, "Know thyself, the kingdom is within you," mean you must know yourself and the Order of the Universe, the dialectical constitution of life itself. (How is it that you were created by this order and by what means was the life force itself brought into being?)

Now you should be able to comprehend that the words of

Epictetus, "Everyone is happy; if not, it is their own fault," are exactly correct. The fault or error is in not having practically realized this dialectical Order of the Universe. False and mistaken education is an invention of the evil minority who are in a governing position. The rule of the people is always in the hands of more yin or more yang groups, each in their alternative turns. If a ruler does not wish to succumb to this tendency and be overthrown by antagonistic forces, the government or regime has only to be chosen with a correct proportion of these opposing groups. But then it would be necessary to establish a new Copernican method of electing leaders.

At last now, you have the key to the kingdom of heaven, the Order of the Universe.

TWELVE THEOREMS OF THE UNIFYING PRINCIPLE

These theorems define the functioning of the relative world in terms of yin and yang.

1. Yin and yang are the two "activity poles" of the infinite pure expansion and are produced infinitely and continuously from the infinite pure expansion itself.
2. Yin and yang, combined in an infinite variety of proportions, produce energy and all other visible and invisible phenomena.
3. Yin activity is centrifugal (dilating) and produces expansion, lightness, cold, etc. Yang activity is centripetal (constricting) and produces contraction, weight, heat, etc.
4. Yin attracts yang; yang attracts yin.
5. Affinity or force of attraction between things is proportional to the difference of yin and yang in them. In other words, the force of attraction between yin and yang is greater when the difference between them is greater, and smaller when the difference is smaller.
6. Yin repels yin; yang repels yang.
7. The nearer two beings or phenomena of like activity are to each other, the more they will repel each other. The farther away, the weaker the repulsion.

8. All phenomena are composed of both yin and yang activities. There is nothing completely yin or completely yang. All is relative.

9. There is nothing neutral. There is always yin or yang in excess. No phenomenon is balanced. Polarization is ceaselessly working and is universal.

10. All phenomena are constantly changing their yin and yang components. Everything is restless. In other words, yin and yang are constantly changing into each other.

11. Yin produces or becomes yang and yang produces or becomes yin at the extremes of development.

12. Everything is yang at its center and yin at its periphery (surface).

The last two theorems are very important and useful, as will appear more and more clearly as you advance in your studies.

"One produces two, and two produces three," said Lao-tsu. The "three" of his saying represents all that exists in this relative world. After oneness divides, creating the polarity of yin and yang, succeeding divisions continuously produce an infinite variety of phenomena. Where one force meets another (yin and yang meet), spirals form, thus producing more and more phenomena. This process is repeated endlessly, everywhere, all the time.

Yin is centrifugality: the force of expansion, dilation, and diffusion. Yang is centripetality: the force of contraction, constriction, and cohesion.

Yang produces heat, light, infrared radiation, activity, dryness, density, and hardness. Yin produces cold, darkness, ultraviolet radiation, passivity, wetness, lightness, and softness.

To say that something is "yang" means that its yang (centripetal force) exceeds its yin (centrifugal force), the reverse being true when we speak of something as "yin." For example, compared to woman, man is more active, compact, and hard. His flesh is actually more brittle compared to that of a woman. Also, the percentage of red blood cells in his blood is higher. These factors (as well as many others) are all indicative of the fact that yang (centripetal force) is greater in men than in women.

The Unifying Principle of yin and yang is nothing more or less than the law of change, the basis of all the great religions. We see it in operation every day of our lives, but are often unaware of it. Night becomes day. Sickness becomes health. Ignorance becomes wisdom ... And all vice versa. If yin did not become yang, then what would? If schoolboys were learned, how could they be taught? Such is the mechanism of absolute justice: the yin-yang law, which governs all phenomena, visible and invisible.

The Unifying Principle can, therefore, be condensed: Everything is composed of two fundamental forces, yin and yang. They are seemingly antagonistic, but actually they are complementary. If you could understand this reality fully, nothing would be impossible for you.

George Ohsawa with his wife, Lima, mid 1940s.

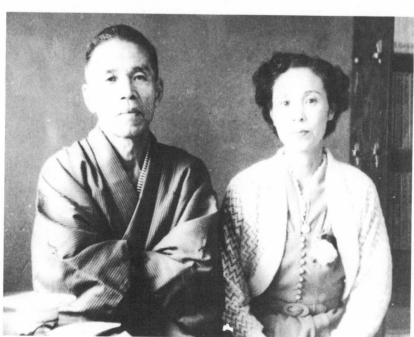

6

THE ORDER
OF THE UNIVERSE

THE ORIGIN OF FAR EASTERN PHILOSOPHY

In order to reveal the unique spirit of the Far Eastern people in its origin and development from the purely philosophic, psychological, and scientific point of view, let us go back several thousand years.

One of the primitive nomadic peoples that had been roaming over the whole continent of Asia settled at an unknown period on the plateau of central China. The plateau is vast, naked, and devoid of humanity for the most part, an ocean of hills and dales melting into the sky at the distant horizon. Sprinklings of hamlets are seen here and there. The sun is setting far off on the high plains.

A man emerges from one of the huts in the central village. His name is Fou-Hi. He is the leader of these people. His figure is massive, solid, and gigantic, like a statue chiseled with a few simple, vigorous strokes of utter precision. His hair reaches to his shoulders. His long beard is black, his nose straight and high, his eyes large, brilliant, and penetrating.

He strides forward with long elastic steps, solid and vigorous as those of a young man. He reaches the terrace, which reveals the view of the entire plateau unto the most removed fields. The wind has ceased over the cornfield from which the moon, full and yellow, rises.

The philosopher-leader contemplates the sky, where the stars have already appeared. This has been his custom for several years. Night progresses.

His age is already beyond eighty. In his youth, he had been the most active warrior, the one worker who knew not fatigue. He had struggled against innumerable difficulties—war with outside enemies, internal strife, famines, great frosts, etc.—and he had succeeded in overcoming them by guiding his people. His fine memory and intelligence enabled him to supervise the agriculture, cattle raising, and other primitive industries of his country. He was familiar with all the needs of their lives. All obeyed him spontaneously with respect and even with pleasure. Later on, when he became the official leader, everyone was satisfied under his rule. Peace and prosperity flourished; it was a golden age. He was able to devote his time to the contemplation of and reflection on all the phenomena of the earth and the universe.

He established the science of astronomy. He synthesized all hereditary knowledge accumulated from generation to generation. He had a rather large group of collaborators and assistants occupied with philosophical and scientific research under his direction.

First, they sought the cause of each phenomenon, which later directed their research into the ultimate cause of all things. They sought it at all levels for years and years. They analyzed everything, criticizing and examining minutely all the results obtained. Their methods were necessarily crude in the realm of experimentation, but they verified their results most carefully and, in the end, deduced a fundamental cause. They then grouped the various causes thus obtained and pursued their induction to the end. By means of intuition and meditation, they sought the essential cause and made efforts to achieve universal synthesis.

The alternating recurrence of light and darkness was first of all considered. The one was a benefactor of humanity, the other its enemy. This regular alternation (coming and going—origin of all vibration), which makes us work, which allows us to rest, which makes the leaves shoot up in the springtime and makes them drop in the fall, was indeed the fundamental phenomenon. The same coming and going, the same opposition was discovered in all of nature. When day ends, the night does not delay its coming. Before night departs, the day is already prepared. Therefore, day is the beginning of night. Therefore, nothing is ever complete, finished; all things are evolving, dependent, and connected. Birth is already the seed of death.

The physical exterior of our existence and the spiritual interior of our life are nothing but one more example of this universal oscillation of opposites. One climbs the mountains and there discovers the factors that distinguish the plain; ocean and land, animals and vegetables, organic and inorganic, hot and cold, fire and water, etc.

The philosopher-leader characterized these innumerable opposites two by two into two separate categories. In the first were found the following relative properties: light, solidity, elasticity, resistance, compression, heat, weight. In the second: darkness, softness, flexibility, fragility, expansion, cold temperature. Always guided by pure intuition, he was soon brought to interpret these properties by their activities, which were far less numerous; that is to say, constriction, weight, centripetal force, on the one hand; dilation, force of ascension, centrifugality, on the other hand. He named the first of these activities yang and the second one yin.

It was perhaps on one evening of this period that we watched him leave his hut and reach the terrace. He was continuing his profound contemplation. Toward midnight, two or three shadows, as roughly hewn and statuesque as himself, carrying enormous bundles of logs, appeared on the same terrace. They were his collaborator-assistants, come to make a fire for their master. The flames were brought to life. The fire kindled and illumined the master and his faithful disciples.

First, the master made a worshipful greeting to the fire. Then they all sat themselves around it. They did not speak but continued their contemplation while gazing into the flames. Night deepened. The bright moonlight illumined the whole meeting place with a bluish mist. The philosopher-leader was looking very intently into the fire, as if he were reading something in it. All of a sudden, he motioned with his head and spoke: "Yang attracts yin, yin attracts yang."

This was the law long sought by him. He explained slowly and at length in measured tones:

> Fire is evidently yang, and it has and must have the following characteristics: constriction, gravity, and centripetal force. In effect it possesses them all. But air, the atmosphere, being yin, as our intuition indeed senses it, due to its coolness, to its dilation, to its eccentric movement, is completely in opposition to the yang fire. These contrary forces cannot but attract each other. The fire, being less powerful and smaller in size than the air, which is infinitely more vast, is attracted to the power above. That is the reason why the flames rise. One activity always attracts the opposite activity, just as day and night follow each other, attracted by one another just as a woman attracts a man. The fire travels up into the air and continues until all its heat finally transforms itself into cold. Yang produces yin; yin produces yang.

By turning his intuition and his deepened reflection to the universal vibration, to the perpetual oscillation of the two activities, he understood necessarily that everything is in motion, eternally, without ceasing, and that this motion itself varies in time in an exact and regular manner. Nothing is at rest in the universe.

He penetrated deeply into the darkness of contemplation. Finally he found that his obscurity was full of substance, the nature of which was comparable to nothing in the world of light, but that it possessed a particular activity that gave forth to motion, and that this activity itself must be pronounced by two opposed activities that attract one another as is shown by all the phenomena of the world. These former are the ultimate cause of the latter.

He went far deeper in his meditation, but only explained himself up to this point. He designated what he sensed at the heart of his metaphysical work by the word *Taikyoku*, which I shall translate not literally, but philosophically by the expression "essential nature," or the "ether-universe before polarization." It designates that which constitutes the entire universe and consequently all the beings in it. For ourselves *Taikyoku* can be understood only in its two manifestations according to the activities yin and yang in their multiple composites. In other words, essential nature manifests itself through yin-yang activities. One can only understand the ether-universe before polarization by intuition; no word can adequately convey its meaning.

The wise one judged it futile for men to penetrate further into their studies since the principle of the two activities suffices to explain the world on all its levels. Therefore, he did not invent any sign to interpret *Taikyoku*, but he symbolized the first yang activity, the positive point of departure of our world, by a quadrangular stick in order to give his disciples a concrete example and to simplify his teaching.

"*Taikyoku* produces one," said he.

Although "one" symbolizes the first yang activity, it must not be considered as the arithmetical number 1. Numbers, which are perhaps the first scientific invention of mankind, had an extraordinarily deep significance in antiquity, especially in China.

"One produces two," continued the sage. Here we understand by "two" the two activities yin and yang; this is the polarization of the ether-universe. These two give rise to all living and inert beings. If we translate "three" as all possible beings, we have then: "One produces two; two produces three; three is manifested as all possible beings." This last sentence was most cherished by Lao-tsu.

In this statement one sees set forth the theory of polarized monism, and the theory of the evolution of the universe and all creation. The yin-yang theory is not ordinary dualism because there is no being nor any phenomenon purely yin or purely yang; all are extremely varied manifestations of the possible combinations of these two activities. The theory of evolution that follows from this understanding is quite different from that of Darwin. If there is a relation between biological beings at the level of the cells, or at the realm of the function of the organs, this proves that the fundamental life force is one and the same; the principle of one life, in effect, is single, unique: It is the oscillations of the activities yin and yang in infinitely varied proportions.

If life is a manifestation of the two fundamental and universal activities, it can produce itself at all levels, be it in the depths of the sea or on a high plateau—of necessity assuming different forms according to the milieu and the time—because any being is its transformed environment, no being existing independently of its surroundings. The living organic creature, as well as inorganic phenomenon, can have as many origins as, and even more than, the species, since the manifold conditions of environment are infinite in reality. . . .

It has been difficult for Westerners to understand the traditional philosophy of the Far East because its utter simplicity was either too difficult or at first glance too absurd and not acceptable to Western mentality (the antithesis of Far Eastern thinking). My lifework, nevertheless, is helping our Western brothers and sisters understand the importance of my thousands-of-years-old dialectics, so practical and so useful in everyone's daily life.

Our concept of the universe needs to rest on a great principle. Such a principle must not only be valid for the finite world, but must be applicable equally to both the finite and infinite realms. Otherwise, it will not be a principle that allows for unification of all domains and that demonstrates the identity of matter and spirit. Our conception of the universe must clearly explain the relationships between health and happiness, between the body and the environment, between body and spirit, etc. At the same time, it should be a principle that allows for the elevation of man's daily existence to a higher level, one that is marked by a healthy, happy, peaceful, free, and ideal way of life.

Again, I say: Our concept of the universe must orient us toward an unshakeable state of health and happiness. This view must be more than conceptual. Concepts are not real life. They are only photographs. The expression "conception of the world" is far removed from what I want to convey. My thought is inadequately translated by the expressions commonly used in Western tongues: "Concept of the World," "Conception du mode," "Weltanschauung," etc. My preference is "The Order of the Universe."

However we say it, the Order of the Universe must be within the reach of all people and be easily understood by all. We must also be able to grasp it as one great overview of the structure and workings of the whole universe. And finally, it must be applicable to our daily lives in a practical way. Otherwise, regardless of how brilliant our theories may be, they will be useless and of no value whatsoever when it comes to curing illnesses.

Perhaps there are those who could think of my conception of the universe as deriving from the Unifying Principle to be somewhat infantile. If by "infantile" they are referring to the simplicity of a child, then it's true that the Unifying Principle fits the description, because its structure is made up of two elements only: yin and yang. It's as simple as a compass, but very practical and useful.

More than one hundred thousand people who have been helped simply by following a macrobiotic diet can testify to the benefits of the Unifying Principle at the physiological level. In spite of this record, there are still an enormous number of stubborn souls who are unaware of the benefits of macrobiotic living. I wish I knew how to convince them.

THE FINITE AND INFINITE WORLDS

From time immemorial, the sages of the Far East, out of their vast perception of the Order of the Universe, have known that our finite, relative world was conceived by the infinite, eternal, and absolute world and is continually nourished by it. They also understood this concept to be the explanation of the source of life.

The following works—the *Heart Sutra*, the *Tao Te Ching*, the *I Ching*, the *Upanishads*, the *Bible*, the *Kojiki*, etc.—all describe systematically, as it were, the Order of the Universe and reveal us to the origin of the world. But modern man does not fully understand what is written in these books.

What is important to understand is the relationship between the material, finite world (the world of man) on the one hand, and the spiritual, infinite world (the world of God) on the other. The finite world, as great and vast as it is, is only an infinitesimal part of the infinite world.

Here on Earth, we are faced with an excess of population; in the infinite world this cannot even be considered to be a problem. Since the beginning of this world, trillions and trillions of beings

Comprehending Life

When George lectured, his English was broken, and he apologized for it. However, when he gave his lecture on yin and yang, it was so simple, a child could understand it. As he explained deeper and deeper, I could see the logic of it. There was much more to it than I had imagined. He wasn't just talking about diet—he was talking about life. He was talking about connecting everything in the universe.

When he finished the lecture, he said, " Are there any questions relative to anything?"

And somebody said, "What about the solar system . . ."

George responded, "Yes, that is a spirallic form," and so forth.

And someone wanted to know the origin of cancer, and he answered him. There were questions about anything you could conceive of, and he answered all of them logically in terms of yin and yang, and very simply. When he did that, it hit me: This is the most incredible man I have ever heard. He comprehends life! In my life, I have known men who have comprehended a certain aspect of life—specialists who know a great deal about one thing. But George seemed to know about everything there was to know. It was then that it dawned on me that I should study this man more deeply.

Alex Lesnevsky
Retired from Chico-San, Inc.

have been born and have died, and all of them have been received into the infinite world. It has never been heard that even one of them was refused admittance. That's another way of saying that the realm of death is also infinite, nothing more than another synonym for the world of eternity, the dream, the spirit.

Such is the Order of the Universe. No reason, though, for taking our own lives, as some do in their anguish and despair over the inevitability of death. Rather, we should have a good time and make our life's voyage as happy as possible. But such happiness is the good fortune only of those who know where they are going, namely, to that land that gave birth to us all. They can have a good time in life, like young people on an outing. They can let themselves run, dance, and sing. Sick people, on the other hand, won't enjoy the trip and it's their own fault they can't. The true cause of illness is desire, which comes from greed, which results, in turn, from ignorance about the Order of the Universe. I, who have counseled some fifteen thousand sick people, say it outright: Desire, greed, blindness of heart, arrogance, and pride—all these are characteristics of the sick. And it all comes from the ignorance and stupidity caused by the cloud that separates us from true wisdom.

By nature, we possess a cloudless wisdom, given that we are born of that infinite, absolute world, which is of God. We are all children of God and citizens of an infinite, absolute world. Forgetting this truth is the cloud that causes us to be sick.

This cloud is created by an education that would have us believe that there exists only this finite, material, incomplete, and ephemeral world. And in truth, all human knowledge is criminal in nature if it does not have as its object the infinite, eternal, and absolute reality, namely, God.

Given that the world of spirit is infinite, flowing, whole, and free of all concerns, we might call it the world of God, of the universe, of the way, of nature. That this infinite and spiritual world has brought forth the finite and material one is beyond proof. Life does not exist without spirit. That's why it isn't easy for us to grasp the meaning of life.

What is life?

No one has ever been able to explain what life truly is in any comprehensible way. I consider life to be a passing phenomenon in our finite, changing world. According to Figure 6.1, it's clear that life comes from the infinite world and follows three stages of development.

The first stage is known as infinite expansion. It is infinity, the world that has no beginning and no end. Other names for infinity include: eternity, the absolute, oneness, God, spirit, nature, the *Tao*, *Taikyoku*, truth, love, justice, freedom, happiness, highest

Figure 6.1 Constitution of the Universe

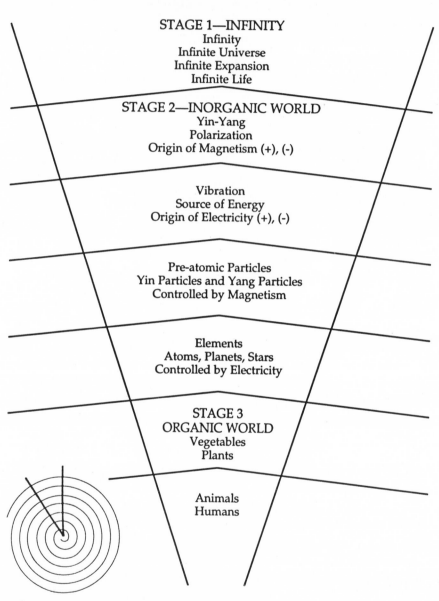

STAGE 1—INFINITY
Infinity
Infinite Universe
Infinite Expansion
Infinite Life

STAGE 2—INORGANIC WORLD
Yin-Yang
Polarization
Origin of Magnetism (+), (-)

Vibration
Source of Energy
Origin of Electricity (+), (-)

Pre-atomic Particles
Yin Particles and Yang Particles
Controlled by Magnetism

Elements
Atoms, Planets, Stars
Controlled by Electricity

STAGE 3
ORGANIC WORLD
Vegetables
Plants

Animals
Humans

This diagram is a section of the logarithmic spiral showing the continuity of the world of infinity with the relative worlds.

will, supreme judgment, and seventh heaven. All analytical, mechanical, and statistical science is invalid in the infinite world. In the infinite world, there is no specialization.

The second stage of life is the spiral. Infinite expansion begins to polarize itself in space and time as a result of centrifugal (expanding) force. The spiral is produced when the branches of polarization intersect and collide. The first orbit of the spiral has two poles: yin (expansion) and yang (contraction). The yin-yang world is the foundation of the relative world. In the second orbit energy is produced, creating the appearance of space and time, dilation and compression, silence and sound, cold and heat, and darkness and light. Thus, this orbit is known as the world of vibration or energy. In the third orbit elemental particles such as the electron, the proton, and all subatomic particles from which these are derived, appear. The subatomic particles may be divided into yin particles and yang particles. This world is known as the world of pre-atomic particles. In the fourth orbit, pre-atomic particles give rise to atoms, which in turn, through a process of compacting, become the stars. That's how the first solar system was born and how millions of solar systems were created in a constantly expanding movement. This is the world of matter, the inorganic world.

The third stage of life begins at a given place and moment in the world of matter. This happens naturally by spontaneous generation. The result is the organic world, a very small part of which is transformed into living beings. The organic world contains two orbits of the spiral, called the vegetable and animal worlds respectively. The vegetal world is the origin of the animal world. All plants have chlorophyll, which makes them green. Take out the magnesium from the chlorophyll, replace it with iron, and the chlorophyll changes to hemoglobin, which is the essence of blood and, in turn, the essence of animals and man. Since the worlds of vibration or energy, pre-atomic particles, elements, vegetables, and animals all come from the world of the two poles (yin and yang), antagonisms always exist, such as those between men and women, life and death, young and old, right and wrong, beauty and ugliness, up and down, high and low, active and quiet, etc., in the world of humans.

In summary, the three stages of life are:

1. Infinite expansion (infinite world without beginning or end).
2. The spiralic polarization of yin and yang, that is, the inorganic world.
3. The appearance of living beings, that is, the organic world.

The third stage of life is what we know as our daily existence in this world. The second stage is the world of death. So death is the mother of life. Life is a passage by which living beings are liberated from the finite world to enter into the infinite world, beginning at the human level, ascending through the animal and vegetal worlds, then on through the worlds of elements, pre-atomic particles, vibration or energy, the two poles of yin and yang, returning finally to the infinite world.

The second and third stages are characterized by changeability and uncertainty; they are the stuff of everyday life, passing worlds filled with illusion. The first stage, however, is infinite expansion without beginning or end, the origin of all life.

We have at last discovered the Order of the Universe. It embraces all since it is the order of infinite space and infinite time. The word "order" carries another meaning: command, directive, instruction. In China that is all summed up in one word: *Ming-Ling*. "Ming" means heaven (yin) and "Ling" means earth (yang). Man is born between heaven and earth, and so must live according to the order of yin and yang. In this world all is subject to change; everything changes. Only the Order of the Universe remains unchanged. It's only natural that the finite world obey this Order of the Universe since the former arises from the latter. This order is extremely simple yet it explains everything in the phenomenal world that can be understood in terms of yin and yang.

Imagine that the universe is a cogwheel of infinite diameter. Materialism may be thought of as the part that projects outward, the tooth, while spiritualism is more like the space between the teeth. People who think dualistically or eclectically can only see the teeth or the space; they can't take in the whole wheel. We haven't talked about the wheel's center, the axis, or about the motor. These we cannot know. Nor do we need to; those aspects we call the infinite, the absolute, God, truth, etc.

Continuing on with our image, we see that infinity manifests itself into the relative world as the yin-yang world. Together they make a first all-encompassing gearwheel that interlocks with a second, called the world of vibration or energy. The two wheels revolve in reciprocal motion, in inverse order to each other (yin and yang). The diameter of this second gearwheel (vibration) could amount to a million light years, but compared to the outer wheel, which is infinite, it would be considered infinitesimal. The second gearwheel is connected, in turn, to a third, the world of pre-atomic particles, a world that doesn't display the great movement that we find in the second (vibration), since the pre-atomic world is yin. The third meshes with a fourth, the world of elements, which is yang, and this, in turn, with a fifth, the vegetable world, which is yin. The sixth and smallest wheel is the world of man, which is yang.

This image may help to describe how the universe is constituted according to yin-yang structure. It is my vision of the universe, of the Unifying Principle; it is my concept of the world.

The Unifying Principle of yin and yang, which is a projection of the Order of the Universe, is very useful because of the following characteristics:

- It provides structure and direction in all domains of life (spirit, body, discipline, technology, theory, practice, war, peace, etc.).
- Everyone, old and young, can understand it and apply it in all aspects of life at any time and in any place.
- It accepts all antagonisms, demonstrates their complementarities and mutual affinities, and includes everything. Consequently, even when someone adopts an exclusive and aggressive attitude towards us, we are capable of staying morally calm and taking responsibility for setting matters right.
- It is found at the intuitive level in the myths of various ancient cultures, even though it may be only in an incomplete and partial form.
- It is the eternal order. There is absolutely no need to modify it. Once learned it will never be forgotten.

We can summarize what we've said so far in the following way: The Unifying Principle is a "polarizable monism," which means that the universe is organized according to the yin-yang order, some examples of which are response, mutual correspondence, complementarity, and affinity. To put it another way, by means of the Unifying Principle we arrive at a global view of all phenomena of life (which are only the natural development of that yin-yang order), thereby receiving a key that can unlock for us a life of health, happiness, and peace, and furthermore enable us to transform every misfortune into a celebration of life.

Another way of saying this is: The Unifying Principle is a vision of the world that is based on the key idea of the unity of matter and spirit.

THE MASTERPIECE OF CREATION

Among all the animals that the infinite, God, created out of vegetables with the assistance of the inorganic world, man is a masterpiece. It could be said that the creation of the other worlds, from the yin-yang world to the vegetable world, are the Creator's sketches. But the world of man is the masterpiece, the ultimate and most perfect.

He who has made up his mind to live in accordance with the Unifying Principle, or universal compass, possesses an infinitely free life, happy forever, and totally just. He may choose any course in the life to come, since he himself is the controller-pilot of the infinite process of transmutation (life).

The orbits of the spiral are not, in fact, concentric. My sketch is wrong and must be a bit corrected. They shape a logarithmic spiral and between them there is no boundary. Should there appear to be a boundary between the seventh heaven (the infinite) and the world of materiality, consider it as imaginary and just for convenience. This logarithmic spiral shows us that our concept of the universe is a polarizable monism. Its origin being the infinite, its speed is infinite too. It leads to man, heir-prince of the heavenly kingdom and king of this world of materiality and relativity.

Curiously enough, all problems, not only medical ones but also social, psychological, scientific, and philosophical ones, can be solved by the use of this spiral. Therefore, I call it "the magic spectacles" or "the new Aladdin's lamp." Here are some examples:

- Where did Man come from? He did not come from his mother, out of a microbe, or, with still less reason, from the ape. But as you can see in the logarithmic spiral, he did come from his foods—i.e., vegetables and their products. All animals are the transformation of the vegetal kingdom. And lots of them are halfway in the process of transmutation between the vegetable and the animal kingdoms. So are all the microscopic beings, including the components of our cells. Our nails, for instance, are an example of vegetable transforming to animal. This transition can be quite a long process, perhaps taking hundreds of millions of years.

- Which came first, the chicken or the egg? The famous philosopher Bergson regarded this question as being absurd and without solution. But it is easy to answer with the logarithmic spiral. Neither can be the first. Both are produced, like man, at the same time by the infinite, with the help of the other worlds, from the second to the sixth: vegetable, elements, pre-atomic particles, vibration or energy, and the two poles of yin and yang.

- What is disease? With the logarithmic spiral, the answer is very easy. Epictetus said: "If a man is not happy, it is his own fault." But there are lots of unhappy people or those who regard themselves as such; few agree with Epictetus. If some of them accept him, they do not understand the ultimate reason for their unhappiness. But I should rather say: "If a man is not happy, it means that, consciously or not, he has violated nature's law, the Order of the Universe, because his supreme judging ability is veiled." (See Chapter 4 on judging ability.) This clouding of the supreme judging ability is often a result of embryological, familial, scholastic, or social education. Why then would the omniscient infinite have prepared such a foolish judgment for man? Is not man doomed for this relative world, ruled by the universal law, "What begins ends"? It is disease that leads us toward health. If one errs in the use of therapeutics, for instance by following symptomatic medicine, this is the starting point for the principles of health. This is the Order of the Universe.

Illness is the very helpful guide that leads us toward an understanding of the constitution of the universe. It is a creation of the infinite. Without disorder, there could be no order. That is why illness as our guide should not be rudely destroyed by surgical operations or with chemical medicaments.

The vegetal is our well-beloved mother, our physiological and biological womb. But what is the origin of the vegetal world—our great biological mother? Everybody knows it: the inorganic world of elements, earth, water, and air.

The inorganic world, yang, is the very mother of the vegetal one, yin. This is why Jesus said on the human level, "Love thine enemies." We must be grateful to our enemy since it is due to him alone that we are as we are. The world of relativity is dialectical. If you have understood this dialectical law, you will be able to realize, answer, judge, predict, or define all things.

Accept everything with greatest pleasure and thanks. Accept misfortune like happiness, disease like health, war like peace, foe like friend, death like life, poverty like prosperity—and in case you do not like it or you cannot stand it, refer to your universal compass, the Unifying Principle; there you will find the best direction. Everything that happens to you is what you are lacking. All that is antagonistic and unbearable is complementary. He who can embrace his antagonists is the happiest man.

It is said that we should have respect for life. But, should this be respect only for human life, which could mean destruction of all beings that are not human? This is not respect for life. One must then know life's true significance: the Order of the Universe, which is nothing other than the ecology of the universe and the ecology of the human body. Those who have well understood that grand concept can live a very long and very happy life; it is quite ecological. All vegetables, all animals are aware of this and practice it; but man does not, for his supreme judging ability is shaded because of his professional education.

To understand respect for life, one must first know life's order and then have the will to practice it in order to realize longevity and rejuvenescence, universal love, and infinite indulgence, without violence or cruelty.

- What is will? This is a big question. But look at the logarithmic spiral. There it is sketched. All that exists in the relative world has a tendency: energy, tropism, thirst, or hunger—this is will. It is the infinite's will—polarized, faded, and colored through the relative stages. Infinite and omnipotent will is the infinite. The greatest will that realizes everything is that of one who knows the Order of the Universe, the infinite.

  If you are anxious to develop your will to the highest stage, you have just to purify your body in accordance with the biological, physiological, and logical laws that I have explained at length in the first chapters of this book. Then, you will become the masterpiece of creation.

SEXUALITY: THE DAYBREAK OF LIFE

Life is a passionate sonata played by the two invisible hands of yin and yang. In fact, it is one of the primordial laws of nature that yin and yang are strongly attracted to one another. Sexuality is the very daybreak of life. It is the basis of all existence—the key to genesis. Even atoms, elementary and nuclear particles, possess sexuality—in the form of attraction and so-called "binding force." All the more so for all living beings.

Love between stars and planets has been called, falsely, "universal magnetism." This notion (Newton's) became the basis of modern physics. Sexuality being the primordial Order of the Universe, all life depends upon it. Neither existentialism nor essentialism (nor any other view of life) could have been born without it. In fact, all living beings, as well as inorganic atoms, stars, and galaxies, possess sexuality. Everything with beginning and end moves in response to its forces.

There are seven stages of love: mechanical, sensory, sentimental, intellectual, social, ideological, and universal. With few exceptions, Westerners know only the mechanical (blind) and sensory

Ohsawa's Confession

At a seminar in Los Angeles, Ohsawa's lectures were brilliant. He talked about transmutation and his experiments that were going so well, and he gave us information on the healing qualities of specific foods. And one night at a campfire (I remember this time when George was almost bald), someone hollered, "Confessions!"

And George said, "Tonight I shall make a confession. . . . The last time I was in America, I was with Tommy Nakayama after a lecture. Tommy said to me, 'I will take you someplace.' I said 'All right.'"

So Tommy took him to a speakeasy sort of place where Tommy knocked on the door and somebody inside opened up a little window and then let them into this private club.

George recalled, "Everywhere, ladies and gentlemen—they are all drinking and dancing, and they are serving chicken. So I decide just to enjoy myself. So I drink whiskey and eat chicken all night—marvelous party. A short time later, I lost all my hair!" And then he started laughing.

Everyone laughed. You know, for such a great man to make such an admission of foolishness—to me it was a mark of his greatness—he could laugh at himself. And yet, there was an education there. Even if you are macrobiotic, there are things you cannot do without an abrupt consequence. In this instance, George had lost all his hair. He was just growing it back when we saw him a year later.

Alex Lesnevsky
Retired from Chico-San, Inc.

stages, and have never even heard of the seven words that describe the various stages of love. Very seldom does one meet a person endowed with love of the highest stage (who accepts everything without question forever). It is this that I most deplore in the West. Every morning newspapers tell of tragic love affairs—all mechanical (blind), sensory, sentimental, or social, all short-lived and culminating in murder, scandal, or suicide. Based on love of money, fame, beauty, knowledge, or power, they result in desperation. Although such ties can bind people powerfully, we should seek love of the higher stages—otherwise our lives are like those of the lower animals, who are incapable of the higher stages of love.

The human being is sexual; life is sexual; to be without sex means death. So it is that France, the country of love, of proper sexuality, attracts many Westerners to its capital. Indeed, foreigners who in their own country never enjoyed passionate love, love which teaches the profound significance and joy of being, fall under her spell, especially in the springtime (yang). In their own country, love is almost non-existent. Four out of five men are desperate for sexual satisfaction, suffering a conjugal life they consider torturous. One out of ten thousand, or even a hundred thousand, really enjoys marriage.

Once upon a time, a very brave American came to France in search of eternal love. He was even prepared to remain in Paris for the rest of his life. His name was Henry Miller. Soon, however, he realized that infinite love, as well as the joys of unlimited sensorial love, were not to be found there, and he was disappointed. Everything struck him as relative, ephemeral, and illusory because he was looking for the infinite and absolute within the finite and relative world. Such quests always end in tragedy: waste of time, waste of life. And such is the magic of sexuality—it provides us with the most amusing tragi-comedies imaginable.

Science, too, looks for "K's" (constants). Until recently, the most sought-after constant has been the atom, the hoped for indivisible basic unit of matter. Lately, however, under the urging of nuclear physicists, this constant has "legally" changed its name to "sub-atomic particle." But the idea that such elementary particles are constant is ridiculous.

Likewise, in this floating and inconstant world, this world of illusion, the source of all human tragedy lies in the demand for changelessness. Our particular failure in the case of sexuality is blindness to the primordial polarization of the universe itself. Indeed, the universe is sexual; it is not asexual. Sexuality permeates everything.

It is impossible to progress from dualism to a monistic view of reality; the direction is backward. Rather we must begin, as does the Bible, with monism in order to explore the dualistic world. In Cartesian systems such as Teilhard de Chardin's, the starting point being dualistic, it is impossible to eventuate in a monism capable of unifying matter and non-matter, known and unknown, illusion and reality, or visible and invisible. Children of "visibility," such philosophers reject all that is invisible despite the fact that their great master, Descartes, discovered the "thinking ego," which is invisible! Memory, judgment, will, and faith—fundamentals of our existence—do exist and are knowable despite their invisibility.

The antagonistic but complementary (monistic) nature of sexuality is a great mystery to our modern god, the scientist, who has replaced the omnipresent, omniscient, and omnipotent but outdated God of former times. All misfortunes, diseases, tragedies, problems, disasters, and crimes result from ignorance of sexuality and its law: dialectic monism.

Since as human beings we wish to lead ever happier, more exciting, and more amusing lives (otherwise, why bother?), we must contemplate the mighty Order of the Universe and its Unifying Principle of polarized monism. To assist in this contemplation is, or rather used to be, the only goal of the Church, but this has unfortunately been forgotten. First the Greek Church, then the Roman, and finally the Western Church are equally guilty of having become ritualistic, professional, and conventional.

Sexuality is the essential secret of life, of existence, of being, of adaptability. It consists of two forces (yin and yang), which are contradictory and complementary. Possessing this key, we can gain awareness of the fact that we are always, knowingly or not, in the kingdom of absolute justice, eternal peace, and infinite freedom.

By all means, enjoy love in the animal fashion, at the first stage of judgment, mechanical or blind. But develop yourself, your love, to the second (sensorial) stage, which, however, always ends tragically. Then raise your love to the third (sentimental) stage, which always ends in hallucination. Hurry along, then, to reach intellectual love as illustrated in the biographies of numerous scientists, the social love of revolutionaries and reformers, and the ideological love of the philosophers. Finally, attain the seventh stage of judgment—supreme, infinite, eternal love where only endless happiness and infinite freedom are seen, felt, and known. This is the goal, and the result, of macrobiotic living.

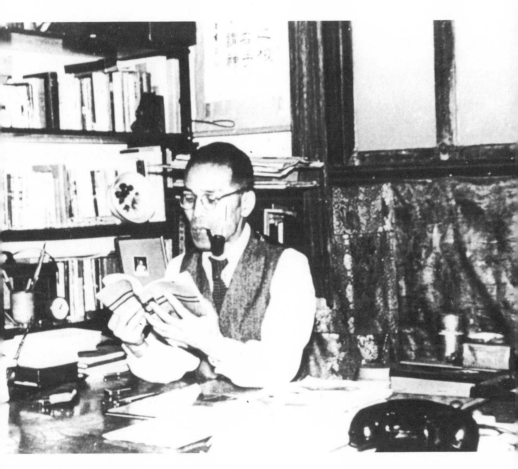

George Ohsawa at Maison Ignoramus, late 1940s.

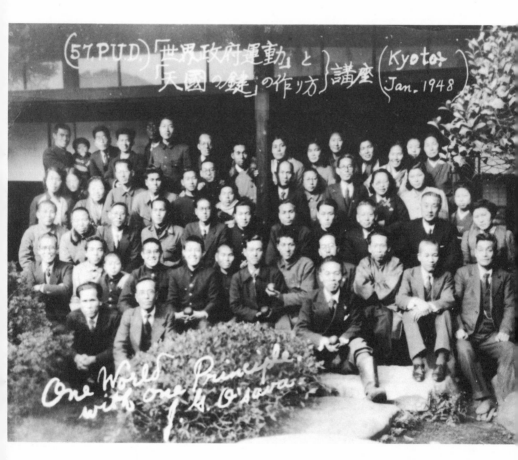

George Ohsawa, fourth from right in front row, in Kyoto, Japan, January 1948.

Part Three

DREAMS
OF THE SPIRIT

The physical life is the false one.
One hundred years of it are as nothing.
It is the spiritual life that is real—
one instant of it is priceless.

George Ohsawa
Macrobiotic Guidebook for Living

7

THE COMPASS
OF HAPPINESS

TWO WAYS TO HAPPINESS

Happiness is the goal of everyone in this world. Happiness was defined by Far Eastern sages some thousands of years ago as a state of being that is determined by five factors:

1. A joyfulness resulting from a healthy, productive, and exciting longevity;
2. The freedom from worry about money;
3. An instinctive capacity to avoid the accidents and difficulties that could cause premature death;
4. A loving realization of the order that governs the infinite universe;
5. A deep comprehension of the fact that one must be "last" in order to become the "first" forever. This implies the abandonment of the goal of being the victor, the winner, or first in line in any situation since the attainment of this goal guarantees one's being "last" eventually. Everything changes in business, politics, science, marriage, in all of life—there is always a new winner. That which is the height of fashion today is out-of-date tomorrow. The man of humility, he who

has no fear of being last, therefore, knows a contentment that is the essence of happiness.

Traditional Far Eastern philosophy—biological, physiological, social, economical, and logical in its scope—teaches the practical way to achieve such happiness. It prohibits the explanation by any teacher of the deep significance of the structure of the infinite universe and its order. The student must discover this significance, the path to happiness, for himself. Accordingly, there are no theoretical discussions, only practical ones. Schools and professional education are considered unnecessary, the makers of slaves. Further, the slave mentality is clearly seen as the cause of all misery and unhappiness.

Remember, all babies are born happy—even the ones who enter into this life blind, deaf, or with some other deformity. They blissfully pulsate in the infinite where disabilities do not matter. It is the parents who are deeply and continually disturbed in the face of what they see as a handicap for their offspring in this relative, inconstant world. They superimpose their unhappiness on the children who are, as yet, oblivious. (The ability to judge relative qualities does not come until much later.) A lack of comprehension of the structure of the universe and its irrevocable order results in sadness for the ignorant parent, not for the child. This is true justice.

There are so many good reasons to be happy. We have air, water, and sunlight in abundance—all absolutely indispensable to the existence of life. They are a thousand times more precious than a diamond weighing two or three hundred carats. We have grasses, rivers, mountains, oceans, and the sky. The heavens are full of galaxies that contain trillions of suns. They are ours! No one can take them away from us. So, merely by token of the fact that we exist, we are the happiest of beings. All living things are so happy—butterflies, birds, fish, microbes . . . they are dancing, amusing, making love . . . If we are unhappy, we are violating the Order of the Universe.

Three factors can assure success not only in dealing with yourself and your children, but also in all of living:

Poetry and Passion

I soon learned that there were three qualifications for Ohsawa's school, the Maison Ignoramus. The student of life must have a dream, poetry, and passion. George Ohsawa loved these three words above all others. "You have to live in these three worlds," he continually told us. "Otherwise, you're dead." His dream of world government and world peace through peaceful biological change permeated every conversation and action. His every comment and gesture reverberated with poetry and passion.

George Ohsawa expected all students to submit to him written comments on what they had learned or were thinking. The first time I submitted a note, it came back with a big "x" scrawled across it in pen. In places, there were holes in the paper, showing he had used his whole strength. I was shocked. I exclaimed to one of the girls, "Never before in my whole life have I received such a grade, and besides, there are holes in the paper."

Fortunately, I did not let Ohsawa's scolding or criticisms disturb me. Being from the cloud-swept mountains, I was used to sudden, unpredictable changes in the weather. Beneath his dragon-like exterior, I could always feel his warm heart. I sensed that he deliberately used humorous and childish ways to educate us. I came to realize that yin and yang really are the compass for a life of health and happiness.

Aveline Kushi
Co-director of the Kushi Institute

1. Study the traditional philosophy of the Far East, applying its Unifying Principle of yin and yang on every level;
2. Practice macrobiotic living;
3. Make many mistakes, for they are your source of learning. Since everything changes, no error is irrevocable; there is nothing to fear.

If you have established good health and have begun to contemplate new horizons of life, educate your neighbors to the superiority of the macrobiotic way to health and happiness, particularly if they are suffering from the same disease as you. If you do not do this, you are not completely cured. You are still exclusive, antisocial, egoistic, and arrogant; you will surely fall ill again.

Exclusivity is both the most difficult disease in the world to cure and the origin of all unhappiness. One must be the sort of person who cannot possibly dislike any other human being. To love is to give and not to take in return. The give-and-take system is a mere egoism, for to give and give more is to become a creator. Since everything you have will sooner or later fade away, to give, give, and give is to deposit in the unlimited bank, the Bank of Infinity. This is at the same time an infinite insurance policy that guarantees infinite life for you. The only premium that you pay is give, give, and give. Give what? Give that which is the biggest and best gift in this world, health and eternal happiness, by means of the key to the kingdom of heaven. And, this key is simply the explanation of the structure of the infinite world and its Unifying Principle translated into the macrobiotic language, the art of longevity and rejuvenation. You can make yourself happy forever by distributing and establishing health and happpiness, by discovering new horizons of joyful, amusing, and interesting living.

Everyone is born happy. If an individual does not continue to be happy, it is his own fault; through ignorance, he has violated the Order of the Universe. If you wish to live a happy, interesting, amusing, joyful, and long life, you should strengthen your comprehension and unveil your supreme judging ability by eating simple and natural food.

In addition, your happiness, freedom, justice, health, and joyfulness must be completely yours. Health or freedom given by others is a debt that must be paid sooner or later if you are not to remain a slave or a thief.

Those who never say, "Thank you"; those who often say "Thank you," but never pay what they owe; those who think that they have paid all they owe by saying only "Thank you" or "Thank you very much" are unhappy. They are more undesirable and detestable than a bandit. They suffer unto the last moment of their lives because their existence is a continuity of debts.

In truth, you cannot pay all that you owe in this life, because you have nothing but what you owe. You will be freed from debt if you distribute infinite joyfulness and thankfulness to everyone you meet throughout your life. This amounts to a real understanding of the structure of the infinite universe and its justice. The Earth gives back ten thousand grains in return for each grain she has received. "One grain, ten thousand grains" is the biological law of this world. He who violates this law cannot live happily.

But, what is happiness in the West? Webster's large dictionary as well as the Larousse and Littre Encyclopedia discuss happiness at length and reach these surprising conclusions: that happiness can never be achieved in this world, that it is a matter of luck, that perfect happiness does not exist on this earth, etc., etc.

My conclusion about Western definitions of happiness is:

1. Wealth
2. Wealth
3. Wealth
4. Wealth
5. Wealth

In short, money is happiness. Gold, silver, fortune, the treasures that Christ scorned have become the most important, precious things in the world. Thus, it is natural that science has become the most important study, that industry is most powerfully active. It is also natural that they could lead humanity into total war. In other words, intellectual judgment has replaced supreme judgment at the head of the list in the West.

I do not imply that intellectual judgment (the fourth stage) is evil. If the West, however, were to reach social, then ideological, and lastly supreme all-encompassing judgment, science itself might produce even more miracles.

The Far East, which teaches supreme judgment from the very outset (considering the other six to be of little importance), has

been totally colonized by Western civilization, as we can plainly
see. In Japan today, sentimentality (the third stage of judgment) is
remarkably well developed.

If you want to know the true nature of a man's judgment, observe
his behavior in love.

Most love in the modern world is either at the first (mechanical
or blind) stage of judgment like that of the amphibious plankton,
or at the second (sensory) stage like that of cats or dogs: It is no
more than superficial, spontaneous, sexual. If one does not have
the emotional strength to live through this blind and sensory love,
one cannot come to that of the sentimental (third) or intellectual
(fourth) stage.

To love is to make one's mate happy. The happiness of which
I speak is really infinite liberty, absolute justice, eternal joy. This
implies loving all—humanity, animals, vegetables. It is the universal love described by Erasmus—love at the highest (seventh) stage.

If you have not tasted the joy of loving one person with all your
heart, with all your might, you cannot imagine the infinite joy of
the love of which Erasmus speaks—universal love or sadness. To
understand, one has to have experienced the unbearable sorrow
of being betrayed by his loved one.

In the spring, one falls in love—the miraculous product of
yin-yang polarization. This should blossom into unlimited, infinite, absolute love. Unfortunately, we arrest this development
and concretize it at the mechanical or sensory stage.

THE HUMAN BOND OF ONENESS

My own definition of happiness is to enjoy doing anything one wants
day and night to the end of one's life, realizing all one's dreams, and
being loved by all during life and even after death. Such a life is
happiness itself. The condition that for me is the great, unique
characteristic of happiness is not that of the Far Eastern definition,
nor that of the West. Summed up, it is to be human.

It is the establishment of free will. To be human signifies that
one has mastered the logarithmic spiral of the Order of the Universe, to which I have consecrated my whole life.

Making Order Out of Chaos

On January 18, 1960, Ohsawa gave a lecture on macrobiotics at the Buddhist Academy in New York City. He randomly gave a list of great men from the East and West and their birthdays. Then he explained the relationship between their birthdates and their characters by analyzing the mother's diet during nine months of pregnancy. He said, "In the wintertime (more yin), the mother eats more yang foods and the baby becomes more yang physically and in character. In the summertime (more yang), the mother eats more yin foods and the baby becomes more yin."

I wrote his lecture including the list of great men in my monthly publication, <u>Macrobiotic News</u>, exactly as he wrote it on the blackboard. He scolded me severely as my article had no orderliness.

I made an excuse by saying, "But I wrote exactly as you lectured."

He replied, "You should always make order out of disorder. Don't be an imitator of others, even me."

For Ohsawa, imitating others is a slave's mentality. He asked his students to make their own opinions and to criticize even his thinking, ideas, or explanations. This makes one free, and freedom makes one happy.

Herman Aihara
Founder of the George Ohsawa Macrobiotic Foundation
and Vega Study Center

The different aspects of this world are due to the differentiation of the oneness aspect of the infinite or absolute. The origin of man is universal soul or spirit, the functions of which are memory, judgment, and will.

The six worlds that manifest themselves from the infinite, non-differentiated world and comprise the relative, differentiated world are the path or way of the eternal, logarithmic spiral through which man must accomplish a voyage in and out.

In other words, the true happiness of man is to explore precisely his native land—seventh heaven or infinity. It is to clearly know the meaning of oneness, to experience the fact that the soul is one, that all things in this world are indivisible despite the fact that human beings are apparently separate from one another and made up of billions and billions of cells. Here is the meaning of unity, the concept of the identity of all humanity, the unification of the entire world.

Having arrived at this point, one cannot distinguish others, and from then on, there is no separation. In the whole world all are reunited in oneness; the term "others" no longer exists. There is neither strife, jealousy, rancor, nor envy. Therefore, if someone experiences the sentiment of compassion or mercy towards others, he is an exclusive dualist and has not fully understood oneness.

Those who breathe the same oxygen, who warm themselves at the same fire, who drink from the same source, who live and nourish themselves on the milk and blood of the same earth, who are born of the same womb, are brothers and sisters. This brother and sister relationship, not a product of law or violence to begin with, cannot be broken by law or violence. Even more strongly so, the relationship between parents and children, between compatriots, between man and wife, between master and disciple, between intimate friends, cannot be broken during the length of one's life. Even if there is a clash of opinions or ideas, at the very most it is a contradiction peculiar to the first six stages of judgment. In the seventh stage, there is no opposition and no need for separation.

In the realm of seventh judgment, there is no possession, no separation, no despair, no promises, no duties, no rights. It is a world without contracts, the world of freedom, the world of the identity of self and others—the soul of millions of individuals. He who speaks in terms of opposition and separation is an opportunist and a dualist. He attests to his ignorance of the absolute and of infinity.

Macrobiotic friends throughout the world; friends who walk

together on the road to infinite liberty, eternal happiness, and absolute justice, who are joined by a stroke of fortune that is extremely rare in this world: Do not separate. Do not abandon one another. There is no reason to discard a friend even if his comprehension is of the lowest sort, because infinite liberty, absolute justice, and eternal happiness are one. There lies the realm of monism. If you abandon your friends, family, or teacher, it indicates that you are venturing into the world of opposition, the world of low judgment and dualism. Never separate, even if you are in conflict and struggling terribly with one another.

A brother is always a brother even after death. If you find shortcomings in your friends, you can help them to change by seeking the cause of the problem. If you cannot make them see the light, your judgment has not yet reached the seventh stage. You must redouble your efforts to improve yourself.

Gratitude is always gratitude—even for a glass of water or a bowl of rice. A debt of gratitude must be repaid ten thousand times over or it will weigh you down forever. You are ungrateful, arrogant, exclusive. Master Ishizuka taught me macrobiotic medicine and rescued me from a mortal illness. Consequently, I dedicated my life to saving ten thousand existences as a testimony of my gratitude: "One grain, ten thousand grains." For me, ten thousand people represent the world. One grain, ten thousand grains is not, in reality, the mere discharge of a debt of gratitude. It is the realization of one's self in happiness, liberty, and justice. Only those individuals who follow this way can become citizens of the land of absolute justice, infinite freedom, and eternal happiness.

FOUNDATION OF ABSOLUTE HAPPINESS

For thousands of years, the saints, the wise, and the scholars have attempted to unravel and elucidate the principle of one riddle, that of love. How does one love and behave so as to be loved like small children? When one loves or wants to love, there always seems to be a contradiction between that love and the freedom that everybody also wishes to obtain and no one wants to sacrifice. It seems the two cannot be established side by side. Parents' love for their children, a man's love for a woman or vice versa, is not necessarily love. This may, at times, be only one kind of sentimentality or egoism. It is well understood that love is a beautiful thing and everyone really wishes to love and be loved and yet, due to the territorial battle between love and freedom, they are in a state of confusion. No one knows how to solve this conflict between love and freedom.

Wise people and scholars of ancient times point out to us very forcibly that the unification of love and freedom is, in fact, the only exit from the problem. They point this out in different words but they are all of the same mind. People cannot seem to understand that the principle of freedom and that of love are one and the same. It is ignorance of this principle that causes all the unhappiness and tragedies of this world. Whence comes this ignorance? It is due to: 1. Bad memory, colorblindness of the memory; 2. Weakened powers of reason, colorblindness of the reason; and 3. The use of timeworn, outmoded, insensitive, and meaningless words. Imperfect words are the product of a colorblind memory and reason. This color blindness has a dominant influence on our spiritual and mental constitution, which is dependent upon our physiological constitution. Just as the function of a machine depends on its physical and mechanical construction, our mental and spiritual functions also depend greatly on our way of eating and drinking, which largely determine our physiological constitution.

Both the quality of our food and our way of eating have changed enormously over a period of thousands of years. In fact, eating and drinking, as well as our environment and way of living, have changed completely just in the last two thousand years. The human function of adaptability, of which reason and memory are only part, has also changed with the ages and with the changes of the human physiological constitution. Yet we cannot return to the method of eating and the foods of two thousand or more years ago. We must create a new method of living, eating, and drinking that is appropriate to our own age and times. This is already long overdue.

But before we can renew our way of life, it is necessary to

Three Thousand Birthdays

I used to be very strict in my adherence to macrobiotic principles and George would look at me and say, "Very bad." Then my wife would go and give him a big hug and a kiss and a big smile. He would look at her hands and eyes and say, "Very good." I could not understand this when I knew she was not at all strict.

One day, I asked Ohsawa why and he said, "She is a very happy and outgoing person and that is very good no matter what she eats. Very strict and serious people will soon fail, and in fact have already failed if they are not enjoying life more each day." On Ohsawa's birthday, he sent us a card from Italy that read, "I have three thousand birthdays every day because to me each breath is like a new birthday."

One day, someone said, "This life is not important because when you die, you progress to a higher plane." George replied, "You only get one body—take care of it and enjoy every minute of your life. Be grateful for every breath you take. Then you will know true happiness."

Dick Smith
Retired from Chico-San, Inc.

renovate some of the outmoded and inappropriate definitions of words that we use for daily conversation and communication. This is much simpler and can be accomplished more easily and quickly than the physiological or dietetic revolution.

For example, one extremely important word is happiness. Absolute happiness means to accomplish all that one dreams (wishes), as much as one wishes, without depending on any tool or implement or help from others. What, then, is happiness in a relative sense? This question is very simple to answer if one grasps the meaning of absolute happiness.

Relative happiness (happiness of this world) is to accomplish what one wishes depending on various aids or tools and within the social circumstances of the age and times.

Absolute happiness is eternal and free, while the other is limited in time and space and is often ephemeral and illusory. Within the likes of a democratic society, in spite of careful thought and consideration for one another, still one may afflict another with a kind of happiness that is, in fact, the root of distress and sorrow for that person. Relative happiness can be purchased with money, authority, cleverness and trickery, knowledge, or ruthless sagacity. In other words, it may be gained through the use of a tool. On the other hand, happiness in the absolute sense can only be achieved through justice and it causes neither pain nor sorrow to anyone. It is inexhaustible and its usefulness penetrates into every aspect of life. The achievement of this kind of happiness may seem impossible at first, but if one truly grasps the compass of universal order, it is, different from Lockean liberty, within our power to actually embrace.

With this compass of judgment readily at hand and prepared for use, anyone can easily realize and maintain all relative forms of happiness as soon as they present themselves. You will have the potential to realize at will both relative and absolute happiness as well as anything else you desire. This compass is an instinctive biologically and physiologically precise tool of justice.

Jesus stated: "To he who has justice, it will be given in abundance, but to he who has not, it will be taken away from him even what he has" (Matthew 25:29).

In the time of Jesus, the word happiness in the relative sense did not exist. This kind of happiness was called unhappiness. Indeed, it was Jesus himself who labelled it as such: "You see all this before you? Truly, I say unto you, there will not be left there one stone upon another that will not be thrown down" (Matthew 24:2). Here, I will once again revive it anew. The word happiness degenerated from that time up to the present day. If your happiness cannot last for a long time, make no mistake about it, it is relative. Happiness limited either in time or space is nothing but unhappiness itself. If you were to inherit the throne of a king and you could do and have literally anything and everything that you wanted for a period of one, five, or even fifty years, and then in the end you were to be guillotined, would you call this happiness?

Jesus said, "For I tell you, unless your justice exceeds that of the Scribes and Pharisees, you will never enter the kingdom of heaven" (Matthew 5:20). The Order of the Universe, our compass, is the justice spoken of by Jesus. You must first possess it in order to enter the land of freedom and happiness. If you possess this compass and are able to wield it freely, you have already obtained the kingdom and you can accomplish whatever you choose for as long as you choose to do so. Now perhaps you can begin to see the true meaning and great importance of adaptability, the real compass of happiness.

If you wish to learn judo, that is, to enter into a *dojo* and study the way of the masters, you must change your view of life and become like a small child. If you can actually do this, you have not only realized the kingdom of heaven, but you are also already halfway towards becoming a master. You have already grasped the most important point. If you continue now, with this childlike, pure state of beginner's mind, to practice diligently and regularly, you will sooner or later gain mastery. The real problem is, how can you—without the aid of any exterior means or device—actually gain, and make a part of yourself, the fresh and wholesome adaptability of a strong, robust, and healthy child?

A little kitten has never gone into the school of judo, but when it is unexpectedly thrown high into the air for the first time by a mischievous child, it knows how to land with its four feet planted squarely on the earth. It knows judo! It is a born master! Indeed, all the animals, including humans, were originally like this. But education has stifled this marvelous adaptability in human beings. Judo is an art and method for reviving this spontaneous adaptability. When a kitten is just a kitten, when it is just born, it has a marvelous adaptability.

All the animals and all vegetables, including even microbes, lice, and fish of remarkable colors in the depths of the seas, have such marvelous adaptability. Giant bears living at the North Pole, sporting and delighting in their marvelous ability, regardless of burning heat or freezing temperatures of 30 or 40 degrees below zero, know nothing of human problems. They never sell their time for money or go off to become soldiers. They attack when necessary and defend themselves bravely and wisely. They are adventurous and risk their whole existence constantly, but they never imitate our stupidity, attempting to destroy their own species as we do with our inhuman bombs. They are much more polite and courteous than we are.

What has become of human adaptability? Has it been lost? Fortunately not. It is, however, in a totally weakened and degenerated state. It often succumbs even to the attack of very adventurous and invisible microbes. These tiny microbes, who are able to kill this extraordinary giant—are they not great teachers of judo?

Jesus Christ, who fought alone against thousands of powerful enemies and, in the end, secured the most final and almost permanent victory, was a champion of judo. I have written of this in Chapter 8 on The Eternal Peace of Jesus.

Napoleon was also a champion, although he had never learned the art that leads one to become an emperor. He lost the final battle because he placed too much confidence in his own power. Kant and Hegel, Marx and Lenin are also remarkable champions. Marx was the strongest, however, because he utilized the power based on the greatest of algebraic functions (distance/time) and minimized the time factor. Ralph Waldo Emerson, Henry David Thoreau, Abraham Lincoln, Benjamin Franklin, Jean Jacques Rousseau, George Bernard Shaw, Anatole France, and Romain Rolland were all great champions and yet some among them died young. This indicates that they did not have time to practice physiological judo or that they were not especially interested in the preservation of health through proper nutrition or diet.

A truly great person is happy. Heaven belongs to him or to her. One who is great and strong does not engage in verbal disputes. One doesn't attack or ridicule. One embraces everything. One doesn't view hardship as suffering, but rather rises above it and uses it for personal growth and improvement. A truly great person is one who, with his or her own intuitive judgment of universal order, unites all the various miracles of life and nature. This is like the tailor dedicated to the making of an elegant suit, assembling all the material and binding it together by concentrated effort. People such as this are pure and seem to be invisible, blending through everything. Their heart and mind are the reality of peace and their total activity is justice and freedom.

This is why I am telling you of a different medicine that is, in fact, nothing more than an application of the Unifying Principle of the philosophy and science of the Far East. This will assist you greatly in perfecting your art and your comprehension of judo's technique and its underlying principle. Furthermore, it will enable you to enjoy practicing for as long as you choose.

Macrobiotic medicine is a physiological art or technique for the realization of the single most important quality, the superb character of a small child. It is therefore the key to the kingdom of heaven. It is a special art that revives one's enfeebled adaptability to become more like that of a kitten.

It is a different kind of medicine, totally unknown in the West until recently. It is an art of rejuvenation and long life; a medicine and dietetic regime that restores youthfulness and freedom. It is a study of health that makes us younger every day without the use of any special treatments or techniques. It is a blueprint for a happy and healthy life. It is extremely practical, simple, inexpensive, and easy to realize for anyone, anytime or anyplace. This medicine has a history of more than five thousand years. It is a physiological application of the dialectic principle of life that has been totally ignored even in Japan since the importation of Western civilization about a century ago.

Now we can answer the riddle of love. To love in the absolute sense is to lead others, born in the midst of eternal happiness and yet unaware of its existence, to trade their insatiable attachment for worldly possessions and their incessant search for ephemeral and fleeting pleasures for the practical realization of eternal happiness. The most practical step towards this is the rejuvenation of our physiological constitution, which is, as we have seen, the foundation of absolute happiness.

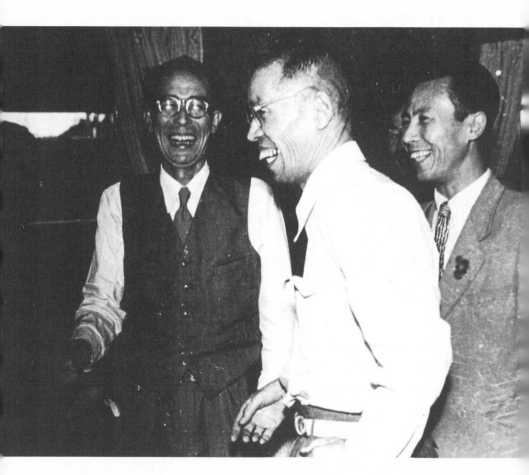

Goodbye party for George Ohsawa, center, as he prepares to leave Japan for India.

8

A WORLD IN PEACE
AND FREEDOM

JUSTICE FOR ALL

Our dialectical and practical medicine can be reduced to one simple phrase: justice for man. This concept should not call to mind the image of the courthouse prevalent in so many Western countries: a square, cold, rigid building, severe-looking from the outside and somber, cold, nasty, and cruel within. Justice, as traditionally understood in the Far East, is joyful, familiar, kind, and amusing. Justice for man comes from absolute justice: all-embracing love, Divine Love. Absolute justice is the impartial law that applies to all that exists. It is the Order of the Universe, which creates, animates, and transmutes everything. It is the spirit of all existence. It is the quintessence of the infinite universe, life. Absolute justice provides everything for us. It makes no exceptions and omits nothing. It gives us "bad" weather as well as "good," cold as well as heat, scarcity as well as abundance, difficulty as well as ease, "enemy" as well as friend.

Absolute justice is absolutely impartial, and he who knows this is also impartial. (However, if you have very strong preferences, it is wiser, in making a choice, to seek a proper balance between yin and yang. In the Far East, it has long been thought that no more virtuous attempt is possible in life.)

Keep Your Promises

The first American macrobiotic summer camp was held at Southampton, New York, in 1960 and lasted for two whole months. Ohsawa asked me, "Cornellia, could you help with the cooking at the camp?" I enthusiastically said, "Yes!"

I attended the camp with my two-and-one-half-year-old daughter and my one-and-one-half-year-old son. My husband, Herman, drove George and Lima Ohsawa to the camp every Saturday and back again every Monday. I stayed at the camp and worked every day with no day, or meal, off. One week before the end of the two-month camp, I vomited a little bit of blood. A few days before this, Ohsawa had asked me, "If you are going to Europe with us after the camp, shouldn't you go home early to prepare for the trip?"

I had responded, "I'm almost finished with my preparations for the trip to Europe, so I can help for the rest of the camp." However, I was shocked when I vomited blood and thought it would be better to go home with the children and rest. I asked Ohsawa if I could go home but he said "no." He knew my condition was not serious.

After the camp had ended, George and Lima returned with us to our apartment in New York City where they had been staying during the weekdays of camp. Ohsawa did not talk to me for a couple of days and this was very unusual. Lima told me to apologize to George for asking to go home early so I did.

Then, Ohsawa told me, "Cornellia, once you make a promise you should not break it, even if you vomit blood. If you break a promise even once, then no one will trust you."

I thought this was very severe, but I have never forgotten what he taught me. It made me appreciate his teachings even more and I have continued to live by them in my daily life.

Cornellia Aihara
Co-director of the George Ohsawa Macrobiotic Foundation
and Vega Study Center

Since we are heirs to the entire infinite universe (life, which includes life and death), we need never kill—not even in "self-defense." There truly is no enemy anywhere in the infinite universe. Cancer, allergies, heart disease, mental illness, crime, and even capitalistic imperialism are all amusements with which our invisible producer-director-instructor (oneness) continually confronts us and thereby reveals itself to us.

There are many things in this world that we "see without seeing," "hear without hearing," and don't understand, even though we speak about them constantly. Justice is one of these. Briefly synopsizing the Encyclopedia Americana, justice is defined as "something like happiness; it can never be attained by man." (This sort of judgment is to be expected from those who perceive only the "visible.")

Justice of man is attainable. But in order to attain it, we must first understand absolute justice. Absolute justice is not only the basis of justice for man, it is the basis of all existence; it is the source of all visible and invisible phenomena. Without it, we cannot live, not even for a second. It is what I call the Order of the Universe. It is everywhere, all the time. If you understand it, you also understand and practice justice for man.

Both "visible" and "invisible" exist, the former measurable in the phenomena of the world we can see, the latter hidden beyond the reach of instruments. The kings of the world of "visibility" are matter, force, and war, while those of the world of "invisibility" are spirit, acceptance, and peace. The goal of the world of "visibility" is relative (satisfaction of desires), while that of the world of "invisibility" is absolute (awareness of oneness). This is why the West and the East have so little in common.

The seventh condition of health and happiness is the complete understanding and application of justice for man. This condition is far more important than the others—so much so that, if it is not fulfilled, achieving the other six is meaningless.

Since about the age of fifty, I have completely devoted myself to spreading the macrobiotic method of curing the body and soul. Pursuing my goal I have often forgotten to sleep and eat. Eventually I arrived at the following conclusion: Nothing is easier to cure than so-called "incurable" disease, but nothing is harder to cure than patients themselves.

Later I realized the importance, the enjoyment, and the suspense that come from struggling against such great difficulty that I have given all my soul and all my strength to the endeavor. Time passed, the earth pursued its course, and I have reached the age of seventy. It is now, at this stage of my life, that I have come to know absolute justice, the Order of the Universe, the source of all spiritual power and "magical" capabilities.

But awareness of absolute justice is not attainable overnight. Body and soul must be trained for thirty or even fifty years. One must climb the steepest snow-slick mountains, bitten by frost at every step of the way. If one is very strict it is possible to arrive at the total understanding and practice of justice for man in only ten or twenty years. But if one depends on a guide or an instructor one will lose one's independence. Self-study is necessary to attain the ultimate goal. The following rules can serve as guideposts on the journey towards the comprehension and practice of justice for man.

- Never get angry. Accept everything with unlimited joy and gratitude, even if it be extremely humiliating, painful, or the cause of great inconvenience. Accept terrible misfortune or deep anxiety with ever-growing thankfulness. Maintain yourself in such a condition that from morning until evening the words flowing out of your mouth reflect infinite gratitude.
- Never know fear. With a mental attitude that is fully prepared to accept whatever happens, seek what is horrible, repugnant, or fraught with hardship.
- Never say, "I am tired; I am in trouble; it is difficult; what can I do?" or any similar expression.
- While eating anything, keep repeating, "What a joy, how delicious!"
- Sleep soundly and peacefully. Never dream, never move. Be content with four or five hours of sleep, awakening with a smile and at the designated time.
- Never forget anything—especially the spirit inherent in the maxim, "From one grain, ten thousand grains."

- Never lie to protect your "self."
- Be precise.
- Like everyone equally.
- Never doubt others.
- Attach yourself completely and solely to absolute justice, the Order of the Universe (change itself, the only constant).
- Discover and contemplate what being alive really means; understand that life is the most precious and greatest treasure in the world.
- Hour after hour, day after day, enjoy the pleasure and thrill of discovering the sublime Order of the Universe.
- Never work, meaning never sell your time or your life for money. Amuse and enjoy yourself to the end. Every day, all your days, live as a free man, the way the birds and the fish do in the skies and rivers.
- Live the principle, "From one grain, ten thousand grains," by distributing joy and thankfulness to everyone you meet.

A GLIMPSE OF INFINITE FREEDOM

The universal concepts that manifest in man's constitution can be expressed as follows:

1. Genuine man has infinite freedom;
2. Genuine man knows absolute justice;
3. Genuine man identifies himself with eternal love.

The one who does not possess infinite freedom is not the genuine man, but a fallen man, a slave, or just a machine that eats. To be free or not depends only upon human will, or supreme judgment. Man is capable of knowing absolute justice. He should not live in any other way. Justice is a necessity. One should not punish a criminal if one is not able to help that criminal understand the constitution of the universe. The fallen man is like an animal willing to distribute happiness to its fellow creatures, but without realizing that its judgment is veiled because it is neither free, happy, nor equitable.

The Infinite Bank

Everybody loved Ohsawa because he loved just about everybody. There were very few people he wouldn't tolerate. He was always a friend, always helping you—that incredible "giving" that is extremely rare. I find that most of us can give only a little. We are not capable of it. We are hung up on one thing or another.

I think George was a free man. He did what he wanted to do. It was Bob Kennedy he told, "In my pocket I have only some change and that is all the money I have. Yet I will spend over a hundred thousand dollars this year." He had no concern for where it would come from. It always came.

He said, "The infinite bank will take care of you—you don't have to worry about a thing." That is, to my mind, infinite freedom.

Alex Lesnevsky
Retired from Chico-San, Inc.

The number of your intimate and faithful friends is a token of your liberty, of your happiness and sound judgment. The one who is able to love all those he meets, who can establish justice where he finds himself, and is always loved by the ones he knows, is really a free man; he is happy and honest.

He who is applauded for being a courageous man does not know courage. He is so completely involved in his courageous action that he has no time to contemplate what he does. That is, he does not know what it is in the sense that we, as observers of his action, know it. Likewise, he who is 100 percent honest does not know what honesty is nor does he who is righteous know righteousness. Further, the healthy person knows not health. They are all humble. Knowledge of one's courage, honesty, righteousness, or health is the identification card of the limited, relative, illusory world, not of the infinite kingdom of heaven.

If you are sure of your ability, quality, power, knowledge, or fortune, you are a prisoner of this limited world. If you claim to know courage, honesty, justice, patience, or health, you have no modesty and in reality you are a stranger to all of them.

Here is the core of the matter: Courage, honesty, justice, happiness, and freedom cannot be given by one person to another. You must realize them by yourself and for yourself. If they depend upon others or upon certain conditions, they are all borrowed and not truly your own. If someone guarantees your freedom, your freedom is your debt. The greater such freedom, the greater your debt.

Happiness, freedom, and justice must be infinite, unconditional, unlimited. If you seek them from others or if they are dependent on the conditions of your society, your debt is endless. Your life is that of a slave.

The modern democracy that issues from John Locke's theory is nice to look at, but in reality it is egoistic, sentimental, and defeatist. It is negative. It has no confidence in man. It defends itself by means of "laws." It fears. And its fear is the symbol of a complete ignorance of the laws of the universe.

Man is apt to become inferior to the animal, but he has in himself the potential to become really human and even divine.

World peace or world federation can only be established on the basis of the understanding of life's constitution, and in no other way. Morals and religions have failed utterly. They have been able to avert neither war nor man's corruption. The reorganization of society is not useless, but it will have only a likeness to freedom. Infinite liberty likes only the impossible, and hindrances of every kind. Infinitely free, eternally happy, and absolutely honest man cannot be created by a social institution.

Freedom is to be found in slavery. Light is to be seen on a dark night; the numberless stars and millions of suns do not shine in the daylight. Wise men are not to be found in a wise country; millionaires are not millionaires in a country of millionaires.

Liberty that is planned and then given to the people in a democratic country is not true liberty at all. The liberty that is safeguarded by law is just slavery. The peace that is safeguarded by law is but a peace established through violence.

Health established with the help of medicine or by some instrument is dependent, uncertain, or begging. Such health is shameful compared to that of all animals, even the smallest. True health can be established only by conquest over bad factors that are menacing your life, without using any violence; rather, by a good cooperative and complementary agreement, a universal solidarity, or a most intimate brotherhood established with all the evildoing factors. The fundamental ideas of symptomatic medicine, which tries only to destroy noxious factors, are childish, primitive, unmanageable, exclusive, and pre-Copernican.

There can be no front without a back, good without evil, beauty without ugliness. The total destruction of antagonism is suicide. Total suppression of ugliness, evil, and slavery means death to beauty, goodness, and freedom. If the international union of the feminist league were to sentence men to death and kill them, that action would become at the same time suicide of the whole female species.

Liberty has its significance in slavery and difficulties. Beauty finds its beautifulness only in the presence of plainness. Freedom is to be found only through slavery. The loveliest lotus flower grows in the dirtiest mud. True health can be maintained even under the most unhygienic conditions. During the war, many examples of this could be seen among soldiers at the front. Happiness can be found at the bottom of misfortune. The safest place to be during a heavy bombing is nearest the target of the last bomb.

It must be well understood that freedom can be found and established only in slavery and in the depths of difficulties. Freedom cannot be distributed, but established only by the person who wills it; this world has been created only for free men. Those who are not free must suffer. The free, strong, faithful, and admirable man lives happily even in the midst of difficulties and violence. Only in the deepest of troubles is he able to display the whole of his unlimited fortitude.

If the absolute, eternal, and infinite world, the seventh heaven according to the logarithmic spiral, is the real world, then this relative, infinitesimal, limited, and finished world must be a false and unreal one. The greatest truth is that this relative and false world is therefore the greatest error in the absolute and eternal world. The same is true so far as good and evil, beauty and ugliness, honesty and dishonesty, faithfulness and infidelity, peace and slaughter are concerned. All that exists in the unreal, relative, and false world is designated by a name that is quite opposite to its nature. Nothing is true, real, or infinite; everything is but illusion. That is why, one day, to the amazement of his disciples, Shinran said: "Even the honest can be saved; why not the dishonest?"

Giving freedom to somebody appears to us to be very beneficial, but actually it obstructs the germination of the faculty of freedom. It is a big crime. If you help some poor beggar, every day, by giving him enough to live on, he will keep begging for the rest of his life. You are making a mistake. Besides, you could not support thousands of poor people. All that you cannot fulfill entirely and forever is but a limited, palliative good. There are many great philanthropists dying of cancer. This means they do not understand the correct way of life according to the Unifying Principle.

All the governments of the world, with the exception of New China, officially recognize only one medicine—allopathic. There is no freedom to choose medicine at present. In few countries can one ask help from any other medicine for his health and life. In a free society, monopoly of any enterprise or profession is admittedly under the control of law and government. But government and law must not protect any monopoly, enterprise, or profession when it concerns man's health, life, education, thinking, eating, and drinking.

If there were a billionaire philanthropist who gave all his fortune for the free distribution of modern, chemically industrialized medications, with deep confidence in this dictatorial medicine, and if this medicine were definitely condemned as useless or harmful (because it violated the law of natural selection), he would be sent to prison with all the physicians and friends who cooperated with him. But modern law does not judge or sentence such responsibilities. If another Jesus were to come into our society and cure all patients through faith, he would surely be arrested, jailed, and sentenced by the law, which is the protector of monopolistic medicine.

We must be aware that it is the same for those who are rich, not only in wealth but in every area: sentiment, sociology, industry, science, medicine, religion, agriculture, and technical matters—if they are not firmly grounded upon the constitution of the infinite universe and its Unifying Principle.

Remember that comprehension and application of my philosophy-medicine not only leads to physical health but also opens wide the gates to awareness of eternal happiness, infinite freedom, and absolute justice. You are even protected against "accidents" since it unveils your extrasensory perception or clairvoyance. Many testimonials of such unveiling exist in Japan as well as in Europe and America, but it is better for you to experience and learn for yourself so that your understanding will be deepened.

Give up everything that is not absolutely necessary to your life for at least a month or two. You will catch a glimpse of infinite freedom, eternal happiness, and absolute justice. You may soon begin to understand why macrobiotic persons are completely immunized from disease. The decision is yours.

THE ETERNAL PEACE OF JESUS

We concluded in Part One that physiological health is the most important basis of happiness. It is the foundation of freedom and equality and consequently of democracy and peace.

There is a beautiful saying in Chinese philosophy, "If you desire world peace, you must first establish peace in the nation; if you wish to establish peace in the nation, you must first establish peace in the family; finally, if you desire to establish peace in the family, you must first of all establish physiological harmony and peace within yourself." In other words, you must establish your own physical and mental health.

A state of physiological and moral health is the single most important unit in the establishment of peace in the daily life of the individual in society and in the world. A peace so established is concrete and lasting. Unfortunately, the way to apply this wonderful principle to the daily life of the individual is not at all explicitly pointed out. The religions of love, of loving and being loved, are one kind of art. They are a practical way of developing and refining one's physical, physiological, and moral adaptability. This adaptability calls forth the extremely important judgment of the instinct that had previously been veiled by acquired knowledge. It is an art of becoming like little children.

Jesus was one great master of judo. He was attacked by thousands of enemies who were much more powerful and yet he conquered them and his victory has lasted nineteen centuries. The Pharisees, the Scribes, the heretics and all those who came after his death respected Jesus even though they were unable to understand him. Even this generation of vipers—the unhappy people of today who are enchained by discouragement and anxiety—has been forced to respect him and his works.

Jesus never used force. He forgave his enemies even when they tried to kill him. He utilized their power against them until finally, in the end, they killed him. In spite of that, it is his enemies who, for nineteen hundred years, have been unhappy and punished by being exposed on the cross of the people's judgment. Jesus, on the other hand, is loved by the people for his nonresistance, nonviolence, and his effortless power. He has been able to give courage, pleasure, peace, nobility, eternity, and tranquility to the great majority of the people for nineteen hundred years, even after his death. His enemies have had only sadness, remorse, hatred, and despair. Who is the conquerer? Jesus, the distributor of eternal joy, peace, happiness, and courage—or his enemies, the generators of hatred, remorse, and sadness? Jesus is eternal peace while his enemies represent anxiety and fear.

"The supreme method is to obtain victory by apparent defeat." These are the words of Sun Tsu. Could this not describe or represent the spirit and deeds of Jesus?

Fear, remorse, hatred, and sadness are the emotions that rule the vanquished. That which gives joy, peace, serenity, and courage is victory. This is the eternal victory of Jesus.

Judo is the way of Jesus. When two forces of opposite direction collide, combat or conflict is born. This develops in two different ways depending on the proportion of yin and yang components.

1. The yang, developed by power and training, serves as a fortress.
2. The yin, developed through spiritual searching, creates adaptability.

The yang fortress created by power and hard training is very limited by the laws of physiology and biology, while the method of battle depending on spiritual searching develops more and more. It is divided into two new directions: weapons (yang) and strategy (yin). Weapons are of various kinds and they range from a simple stick or stone (yang) to firearms, among which the atomic bomb (yin) is the newest. Weapons all fall under the category of force (yang).

Strategy also develops in two new directions: The yang type ranges from the simple maneuver to the very complicated strategy of Lenin, and the yin variety is much less visible and more spiritual, ranging from espionage to the philosophical strategy of Sun Tsu. Sun Tsu's strategy was aikido rather than judo; it is continuing to develop even now. Its supreme pinnacle is the strategy of Jesus. In this sense, *aiki* is another narrow gate that leads you to the country of life, the kingdom of heaven; or, in other words, to the universal country of peace and freedom.

Whether one enters by the narrow gate of Christianity or by another way, the important thing is to gain understanding and put it into practice for the development of your physiological adaptability. This is why most people cannot find the narrow gate and believe that it is foolish to seek it. They are unaware of how to make use of their eyes and their ears so that real seeing, hearing, and understanding can become a possibility. Otherwise, how can we obtain the powers of reason and comprehension, memory, and judgment?

If you do not have these marvelous qualities of instinct, you have only to restore your physiological constitution. Without this, all is impossible for you.

In this finite, limited, relative world, there are two antagonists at all levels: yin and yang (centrifugality and centripetality), woman and man, cold and hot, darkness and light, death and life, sadness and joy, hatred and love, spiritual and material, weak and strong, back and front. Man becomes a dualist when he observes these two sides to phenomena without seeing their unity. Antagonism is found at each of the relative stages of judgment: mechanical, sensory, sentimental, intellectual, social, and ideological. In reality, these antagonisms are the "heads" and "tails" of the same coin. Extremes of antagonisms "touch" each other and commingle. One kills his lover at the extreme of love! While this appears contradictory, it is just such contradictions that animate the world and from which man struggles at all cost to save himself. Most men end their lives still puzzled by the enigmas of existence.

Consider, for example, wealth and fame. For years men desperately seek them. Finally succeeding, they awake one day to find their dreams shattered. They have become slaves of their own wealth, are threatened with assassination, attacked because of high reputation, or victimized by a jealousy their own success has aroused.

To understand and enjoy such contradiction, one must unveil the supreme judging ability. This is the explicit purpose of traditional Far Eastern philosophy, with its concept of polarizable logic that has been totally ignored by most of the Western world for nearly two thousand years—in spite of the fact that the Celtic civilization was based on it. Modern civilization, which has colonized nearly all the world, is based on formal logic: relative, conceptual, and materialistic. All exclusive and therefore alienated mentalities belong to this group, seldom if ever freeing themselves to grasp the concept of monism. All who see or believe in only one side of the coin (good or evil, body or soul, sentimental thinking or intellectual thinking) are dualistic, exclusive, and quarrelsome. Only those who see that the two sides of all phenomena, visible and invisible, are front and back or beginning and end of one reality can embrace any antagonistic situation, see its complementarity, and help others to do the same, thereby establishing peace and harmony. All who are quarrelsome, all who find anything intolerable in this world, are dualists. And as long as they remain so, they will never know peace.

LIVING IN PEACE AND FREEDOM

In certain countries, the average age of the people is increasing, according to statistics. But if they are not happy, if they are hemmed into a rigid society, full of fears, beset by anxiety and loneliness, what is the value of a long life? This is the condition of a prisoner with a life sentence. Crime is one barometer of the physiological health of a civilization or culture. A truly healthy person does not intentionally commit crimes. Crimes indicate serious illness. Social solidarity is in danger. This means that the leaders of the society have some grave maladies: moral myopia, spiritual colorblindness, educational schizophrenia, and social and psychological sicknesses. All of these are very difficult to diagnose or even to discern, much less actually cure. The consequences of these maladies reverberate throughout society; if the leaders are spiritually sick, there will always be many sick people in society as well. Social disorder inevitably leads to complicated and grave physical sicknesses of the liver, the heart, and the kidneys.

If the statistics of a country show a high percentage of divorce, according to the words of Epictetus, this is an indication of a generally unhappy society. They do not possess the principle of harmonious unification with which to establish a concrete social solidarity.

The more a police force is necessary, the more a society—as well as the individuals who are the units of that society—has no real affinity, no real connection or bond, with freedom. The more doctors and hospitals there are, the more sickness there is. Freedom is the physiognomy (revealing character) of a healthy society.

If someone were very strong in judo but suffered from spiritual naivete and nearsightedness, that person would be very unhappy. Such a person would eventually be scorned by society. It is the same in the case of a country. No matter how powerful a country may be, if it is lacking the principles, such as justice, that lead towards prosperity and happiness, it will soon witness the sad spectacle of its own destruction.

As Jesus said, "Seek first the kingdom of heaven and its justice." The "kingdom of heaven" is a happy society in which

The Key to World Peace

I first met George Ohsawa at his house in Hiyoshi, Japan.

"What are you doing?" Ohsawa asked me.

"I'm studying world political problems—world government and world peace," I replied.

"Have you ever considered the dialectical application of dietary principles to the problem of world peace?" he asked.

I was puzzled. I was a very diligent student but had never thought about that. Political science, and even social science at large, except for some esoteric cultural and anthropological studies, never addressed the dietary practices of the human race. What possible relationship could food and peace have?

"I never thought of that," I admitted.

"You have to study the relationship between food and human destiny," he said, smiling. "Someday, you will find that this is the key to world peace. Every week, please come and eat with us."

It was not until many years later after travelling to the United States and observing society around me, especially changing environmental and dietary patterns, that I understood the relationship between food and world peace that Ohsawa had talked about. We create the future on the basis of our day-to-day way of life, including our way of eating. When the environment changes, we change. When eating changes, we change. Thus began my true understanding of the Order of the Universe and the practical application of yin and yang.

Michio Kushi
Founder of the Kushi Institute

everybody enjoys freedom and justice 100 percent. Justice and freedom are really the same thing, for justice is the key that makes all antagonisms become complementary.

A society with limited freedom (for example, the four freedoms as spoken of by President Roosevelt) is nonsense. The more this kind of society exists, the less there is of real freedom. I suppose you can imagine a society where the people have the four freedoms but can you imagine a society with four hundred freedoms? After all, real freedom is oneness. If that oneness of freedom is divided, it is proof that there is no understanding of it at all. This shows that its beginning, its growth and progress, its purpose, its value, its mode of existence, and its function are not understood.

Where is your freedom recorded? When and by whom? How much did it cost you? Without knowing all the conditions of freedom, one does not have the right to insist on it.

Judo, like all other valid schools of the *do*, is for the purpose of researching oneself and resolving the enigma that has tormented human beings since ancient times: What is the human being?

This has been a great enigma for humanity since ancient times, a kind of invisible sphinx for those who cannot respond to this question. All animals, even a single microbe or a single animal or vegetable cell, live in total freedom. We are one kind of animal and yet we are almost totally ignorant of the practical dialectic that is the principle of freedom. Freedom being only another word for peace, humankind is unable to live in peace. The complete freedom and happiness of all animals and vegetables living in peace can't even be compared to us. They are sometimes attacked by their natural enemies of another species and yet they never try to injure or harm their own. They have no need for atom bombs or sophisticated weaponry. According to the opinions of Fabre, Maeterlinck, Seton, and others, they are far more moral and, above all, more honest than humans.

Peace is a state of society or world in which one lives in complete freedom without afflicting others. Freedom is the way of living in which one does whatever one chooses and one's actions are appreciated by everyone else also. This is accomplished without the need for any arms or instruments whatsoever and can be realized peacefully in any kind of society.

Individual peace is the spiritual quality of the person who

knows that all antagonisms are also those very same complementary factors which govern over and perpetuate the universe.

World peace is a state in which a worldwide federation leads the people to, or helps them discover the way to, enjoy complete freedom without interfering or causing any disturbance in the lives of those people. This world federation governs and directs the whole society towards the establishment of a more and more elevated culture and it does this in accordance with the principle of life—that very same principle that unifies, guides, judges, and corrects all philosophy, ideology, science, and technology. This is a universal concept, the principle of principles, the dialectical concept of the universe, or more simply, the Order of the Universe.

War is a reaction inevitably produced between two countries where the leaders strive to annihilate or exclude others or take up arms to preserve their wealth or monopolize their assets. Neither the leaders nor the people of such countries are aware of the dialectical concept of the universe, the key that makes antagonisms complementary.

The value of the true judo or aikido is in learning how to live a free and happy life, how to avoid dangerous situations, and how to have the dialectical principle of the Order of the Universe at one's beck and call.

Two or three years ago, a champion American wrestler, a Mr. M., came to Japan to study judo. He could not find any judo champion able to defeat him. Finally, he went to the aikido *dojo* of Master Ueshiba; the master defeated him effortlessly. From that time on he attended the *dojo* daily for the remaining forty days of his stay. He was staying in a first-class hotel, The Imperial. For this Western wrestler, Ueshiba's *dojo* seemed a very shabby place. One day he said to the master, "Master, come to the United States, you can become a millionaire. There is no need for you to live like this." The master paid no attention to him whatsoever. He was in peace and freedom. Or perhaps it should be said that peace and freedom were in him. He had no desire for anything more than his present situation. In spite of his forty days of strenuous training, the wrestler nevertheless left without understanding the attitude of the master or the principle behind it. The deep ideology behind the schools of the *do* is altogether too foreign and incomprehensible for one who knows only the way of force.

Quite the opposite of modern Western arts, aikido does not use much physical force. It is a technique of protecting oneself without the need for any weapon and it employs the least possible physical force, much less still than judo. Some masters of judo are heavy; in fact, it seems that their body weight increases proportionately to the amount that they practice. The masters of aikido, however, tend to be rather lightweight and of smaller stature. It is an art that lends itself very well to women as well as men and to older people just as well as to the young. It is even possible to begin one's practice at sixty years of age or more. I have explained the principles of judo and aikido in order to show their fundamental relationship to the basis of happiness, justice, freedom, and world peace.

Of course, there will always be those who will protest, saying that there is no one who can accomplish world peace. Yet it is not only possible, but for whoever understands the principle of life—the grandiose world view of the infinite, dialectical construction known as the Order of the Universe—it is quite easy. From this view our world, nature, and the whole of humanity is only a tiny geometric point within the infinite sea of consciousness. Therefore, I repeatedly advise you, first of all, to endeavor to truly grasp the meaning of what is meant by "the Order of the Universe."

For those who can accomplish all their dreams completely and forever without the need for any special implement, war never did, does not now, and never will exist. These are the ones who never meet any person they do not like. They are the ones who are always loved by everyone, everywhere.

9

NOURISHING THE SPIRIT

GRATITUDE FOR SICKNESS

I have almost never met an illness that has resisted cure by way of macrobiotic practice—its healing power has amazed me time and again. All patients become well, and especially those who are most seriously ill.

After many years of experience, however, I recognize one ailment as being truly unique and difficult to handle. It is one from which most people suffer. If this ailment is not overcome completely, the patient is always a potential victim—he becomes ill again and again.

Not too long ago, I sent out about three hundred inquiries to people whom I had helped through my teaching. The inquiry included a stamped, addressed answer card printed as follows:

_____ I have completely cured my sickness

_____ I am partially cured

_____ I have quit macrobiotic practice

The recipient of the card had only to check his answer and write in his name. After two months, I had received only one hundred-nine replies.

Here is the disease that plagues two out of three people—the most difficult of all maladies. Although it might be called idleness or stubbornness, it is nothing more than arrogance. Its victims know no gratitude or thankfulness; they miss the excitement and joy of living. They live a sad, dark life. They know no happiness— only coldness and living death. They always complain and give nothing but trouble to others. Even a dog expresses joy when he sees a friend or his master, but these people never emerge from the darkness. They become sick again and again, and usually die early.

I was once consulted by a woman who had been suffering for ten years. Macrobiotic living gave her the help she had not found anywhere else. One year later, she came back to see me and said, "I have forgotten my sickness since my consultation with you. I have forgotten what sickness is. My suffering has disappeared completely."

The fact that after her recovery she did her best to teach others the method that had cured her reveals at least a bit of gratitude. The average person never returns or expresses thanks. He forgets about everything as soon as his pain is gone.

Those who know true gratefulness never forget that they were once ill; they always remember who or what healed them and are eternally thankful.

The most difficult person to cure is the arrogant one. He is the egoist who knows no joy and who does not mind bothering others as long as his needs are satisfied, the man who lives but has no real life.

Unless we cure this fundamental illness, it is useless to consider anything else that might trouble a patient, for such a person can never be happy. If I cannot change him, I have no right to teach macrobiotic philosophy; better that I give it up. Many people think to themselves, "I am healthy," or "I understand." They are the worst offenders, the sickest; the man who is certain that he is wise is actually the stupidest.

Macrobiotic living can be summed up as the way that gives happiness and thus cures such arrogance. This, not the elimination of specific disease, is our aim.

True Appreciation

One evening after a lecture, a friend invited me to a restaurant, saying that she was dying to have a piece of apple pie and a cup of coffee. I was so turned on by the lecture George had given that evening that I felt like starting a very simple diet right away, so I said "no." The next morning, she called to say who should be seated at the counter eating pumpkin pie and drinking coffee, but Ohsawa. He asked her to join him, smiled, and asked her what she would have, telling her to order anything she would like. Yes, you guessed it, very demurely she ordered dry rye toast and a cup of tea. When her order was served, she put some salt on her toast and quietly chewed and chewed her dry, salted, rye toast (while thinking about apple pie and coffee, no doubt).

The stories about Ohsawa range from the wild and the ridiculous to the hilarious and the woolly. He was all of them, and then some. Most of all, he was a man of humor, understanding, love, joy, and gratitude. For many of us, coming from lives that were sadly lacking in expressions of appreciation and gratitude, it was difficult to fully appreciate how great the gift he gave us, and how deep should be our appreciation and gratitude. After eleven years of macrobiotics, I am just beginning to discover what it is to feel gratitude, and now I know Ohsawa in a way I never could experience him before. So, I say, thank you George Ohsawa for giving me, and us, so much.

Barbara Grace
Contributor to *The Macrobiotic* magazine

Our search for health and longevity begins either when we fall ill or after we reach the age of forty and begin feeling weakness. Sickness and weakness are necessary in this world. It is through our efforts to change them into health that we learn gratitude. How dull life would be without the challenge they present.

A great scholar named Toju Nakae, the Saint of Ohmi (a

province near Kyoto, Japan), was scolded often by his mother during his youth. He usually accepted the scolding obediently, without protest or complaint. On one particular occasion, however, he burst into tears. "Why do you cry?" his surprised mother asked. "Because your scolding has become weak," he replied. "It tells me that you are getting old and I am very sad."

The parents of this sort of child have much cause for happiness—he will be an important man as a direct result of the strict discipline with which he has been raised.

Scolding by our parents is part of our training for life and we should look up to them with gratitude for it. Either we get this training from them when we are young or from life itself later on; we cannot escape it, nor should we try. By the same token, we should not attempt to side-step the scolding of God—sickness. It is this punishment that causes our minds to seek Him out.

To overcome sickness by means of injections or operations is to evade God's punishment or scolding. Just as we should be sad if our parents have died and there is no one to scold us, so should we be sad if we do not get sick. We must be grateful for it; if we hate it, we reveal our egoism and cowardice.

We must accept everything given by God with pleasure, including sickness. In winter we must enjoy cold, in summer heat. Animals in their natural environment accept nature as it is without using artificial means to change it; as a result they are healthier than man. Man in his search for pleasure and comfort finds only weakness and disease. To forsake artificial civilization and return to nature is to find the macrobiotic way of life.

This year, I developed a sore throat after staying too long in a warm, heated room. I took no treatment because this suffering was a warning that let me know that my body had become weakened. As long as I am suffering, I am careful with my eating and drinking habits. For this very reason, I avoid treatments. Surely, you see that with this attitude, even if you have a sickness, you are not really sick.

It is more important to reach a similar level of understanding or state of mind than it is to learn to apply any treatment, no matter how effective.

In your attempt to practice macrobiotic living, you may encounter many difficulties. A place to buy the food may not be readily available; if you find the place to buy, the price may be too high; your family, friends, community, society, or the whole world may be against the idea.

In any event, do not worry. The first task that faces you is this one: Understand the principle. You can then apply it no matter what the difficulties may be.

Animals, birds, and flowers live macrobiotically without money. Study and think about them and their lives, about primitive peoples, about the experiences of Robinson Crusoe. Look at the world around you; there are innumerable sources of encouragement and hope upon which to draw.

If you have allowed yourself to believe that your illness is incurable, that there is no hope left, you will not be able to summon up the energy for such investigation and work. Your drive is gone. You are defeated, you have conceded the victory, you have given up the ship; you had better stop living. Even if you live a long life under such circumstances, you will be half asleep anyhow. Human life is not much when compared with the universe, and we did not come here by our own will, so why cling to it so hard? No matter how long we live, we must die sometime; we all leave this world eventually. We are only passengers on an express train called Earth, and when we reach our destination, we must disembark.

For those who practice macrobiotic living, it is not much different. Suppose they manage to live for one hundred years; that length of time, too, is only a second compared to this life of the universe.

Achieve this kind of understanding and free your rigid mind. Then you can live. Without a free mind, you die very quickly. With it, you can study and think. You will have something to do. And with something to do in this world, we can live; with nothing to do, we die. Idleness is a killer.

The individual who no longer has a rigid mind has found freedom. He has given up his vice-like grip on his own mind; he has given up the prerogative, the illusion that there is a freedom of choice; he can freely accept the decisions of nature. Life can be so easy. Refuse to let go and you are a person drowning; the more you struggle, the faster you sink.

Nature . . . she brought us into being, she has nurtured us. We are obligated to humbly and gratefully obey her. When it is time to die, we die. If it is not our time, Nature will preserve us by showing us the way.

Whoever cannot practice macrobiotic living because of poverty is very fortunate and has cause for much happiness. Difficulties of any kind will make him the happiest of all men because he will have more to be grateful for when he finally is able to follow macrobiotic principles. He who is able to practice macrobiotic living with ease cannot easily know gratefulness. The poor person is grateful for a penny. The millionaire is never grateful; even a gift of one thousand dollars leaves him unimpressed. So, he who has more difficulties is more happy. His gratitude makes him happy and healthy.

He who says, "I cannot practice macrobiotic living" does not understand it fully. But suppose that we observe macrobiotic practice to the letter, repeating everything that we have heard like a phonograph. We are still not really following macrobiotic principles. We must reach the point where we can eat anything without fear of losing our health and happiness. We must control our lives by ourselves. If we adhere to a diet that has been devised by someone else, our lives are not our own. We must not be rigid.

Here is a striking example of what I mean: A mother once came to me for some advice regarding her sick son. I suggested a diet for him to follow and he recovered his health. Years later, I met him again—a small, very tense boy of dark complexion. I inquired as to what he had been eating. His mother replied that she still fed him the very yang (contractive, rich in sodium) diet that I had advised six years earlier when he was ill. Although he had been healthy for most of the six years that I had not seen him, she had mechanically continued to feed him food designed for an invalid! The result was that this boy became overly yang. He looked just like the *kinpira* (sliced, sautéed carrots and burdock root) that he had been eating for six years—small, dried-out, shrivelled. This is the end result of macrobiotic practice that has been mechanically applied with no knowledge or understanding of the basic principle involved.

Without a basic principle to follow, any sort of practice is no more than superstition. The principle (spirit) of macrobiotic living lies in recognizing, experiencing, and understanding nature. This is *Tao*—the return to and contemplation of God.

PRIMITIVE MENTALITY

The primitive mentality is without doubt, simple, childlike, and sometimes even ridiculous. But it possesses something that is very beautiful, very practical, and very profound. The fundamental philosophy of the non-civilized primitive peoples is very simple: Accept everything gratefully and without the slightest protest. This is true modesty: unconditional humiliation; the "self" recognized as small, ignorant, dishonest, greedy, and miserable. Without such understanding, no human being can attain awareness of the true self (oneness). On the other hand, the "civilized" people I have met, almost without exception, have considered themselves great, wise, honest, generous, and happy.

To accept everything humbly and unconditionally is to express confidence in absolute justice, which does not bring us sickness and anguish to torment us, but to reveal to our limited understanding the errors we have made in our ignorance. "If a man is not happy it is his own fault."

Gratitude and faith are virtual synonyms. Gratitude is deep joy and faith is deep confidence. He who does not feel and express complete confidence in absolute justice is ignorant, and ignorance is the cause of all disease, anxiety, and "accidents."

How faithful the "primitive" peoples have been to the teachings of Jesus: "Blessed are the meek" . . . "Turn the other cheek" . . . "Love your enemies" . . . etc. And how quickly they have lost their lands to the conquering whites. But I advise you this, my dear friend: Imitate these primitives. Gracefully give away your home, your land, even your country. You will lose nothing at all. And if new "civilized" men come from Mars and ask you for the Earth, give it with the greatest joy. You have nothing to lose, because you

Primitive Mentality

During the winter of 1942, I attended a seminar during which Ohsawa lectured on primitive mentality. He said, "The real cause of Japan's involvement in the world war is an antagonism between Western scientific thinking and the Far Eastern primitive thinking. Since the two concepts are opposite, they attract each other but because they are opposite, they cannot understand each other and this causes fighting. This war will eventually lead to a better understanding of each other."

As an example of the primitive mentality, he told a story written by Levi Bruel. "According to primitive mentality, something that happens in a dream is reality. For example, one day an old farmer in a primitive country said to his neighbor, 'I had a dream last night in which you stole one of my squash.' As soon as the neighbor heard this, he went home and brought back two squash for the old man and apologized."

Upon hearing such a story, some of the audience started laughing. Then Mr. Ohsawa said, "Some of you laugh about thoughts of primitive mentality. However, much of traditional Japanese thinking is primitive. For the primitive mentality, the dream world is Infinity or Reality and, therefore, it is the world of truth. On the other hand, this finite world is a sensorial and changing world. There is nothing eternal here. Therefore, there is no eternal truth here. For this reason, the primitives believe things that happen in dreams are real. However, civilized people believe only what they can see, which is changing all the time. Therefore, they developed science in an attempt to discover something that does not change."

Ohsawa's lecture on primitive mentality gave me great inspiration and insight on life and I became interested in further study of his philosophy. My life was changed forever.

Alcan Yamaguchi
Former owner of the first macrobiotic restaurant
in the United States

cannot lose what was never yours in the first place. Everything you call "mine" will eventually be lost to you, for there is nothing permanent in this constantly changing world—nothing, that is, except change itself, the only constant.

Give everything, and ask for nothing, because everything you have has been given to you, including your life.

REALIZING YOUR DREAMS

Rarely do we encounter men or women of agreeable temperament. The vast majority of them do not know how to attain good humor, yet they are not to be blamed: They are sick. They know neither what nor how to eat or drink. If you are truly conscious of the wonderful structure of the universe, you should be full of infinite joy and gratitude. And you cannot help but share this joy and gratitude with others. Give good humor, a smile, an agreeable voice, and the simple words, "Thank you," under all circumstances and as often as you can.

In the West one says, "Give and take"; in the Far East we say, "Give, give, and give, infinitely." You lose nothing at all by imitating us for you have received life itself—the whole universe—without paying. You are the unique son or daughter of the infinite universe; it creates, animates, destroys, and reproduces everything necessary for you. If you know this, everything will come to you in abundance.

If you are afraid of losing your money or your property through the practice of the principle of "Give, give, and give," you are sick and unhappy, a victim of oblivion. You have entirely forgotten the origin of your fortune and life, the infinite universe; your supreme judging ability is partially or totally eclipsed; you are unable to see the grand order in nature.

If you give someone a small or large part of your fortune, do not consider it to be an application of the Far Eastern principle, "Give, give, and give, infinitely." You are applying here the idea of "give and take," the basic Western economic theory used as a device to justify the violent colonization and exploitation of all colored people. Many so-called social workers, probably the worst offenders in the West, give only the fruits of exploitation and begging. To give that which you have received from others is not at all a sacrifice. We are reminded of Ali Baba who gave only that which he had originally stolen from forty thieves.

The traditional Far Eastern concept of giving, by contrast, is sacrifice, an expression of infinite gratitude and the realization of self-liberation, of freedom from all debt. To sacrifice means to give the biggest and best thing we have. Sacrifice is an offering to the eternal love, infinite freedom, and absolute justice of life. Real sacrifice is the act of joyfully giving our life or giving the omniscient, omnipotent, and omnipresent principle of life. It is *satori*— self-liberation.

Mother Earth gives herself to feed the grass, infinitely. The grass gives itself to feed animals, infinitely. The animals give life to make this world joyful, happy, and interesting, year in and year out. But the human being kills and destroys everything. Why does man not give himself for others? In creation, one dies and is transformed into new life. Man, in his turn, should give of himself to realize the most splendid miracle of creation: infinite freedom, eternal happiness, and absolute justice. Those who cannot understand this are either slaves, sick men, or mad.

If you are cheerful, beloved by all people everywhere, always giving to others of the biggest and best thing in this world, you will become the happiest of all—the one in a million able to express the greatest joy.

By observing my macrobiotic directions, you can achieve all this. You can actually find the new utopias called Shangri-La and Erewhon of which man has merely dreamed for thousands of years.

Macrobiotic medicine is in reality a kind of Aladdin's lamp, a flying carpet with which you can realize your fondest dreams. But to achieve this, you must first of all re-establish your health and gain at least sixty points as outlined in the Seven Conditions of Health beginning on page 35.

Give everything, with greatest pleasure and thanks. Give and give, without mental reservation. But if you give that which you have plenty of and that which you can replace, this is no true gift.

To give really means depriving oneself of what is dearest to one, the necessary and the most important: one's life. Is this then a sacrifice? The word "sacrifice" itself points to a most wonderful concept that is generally admired and seldom practiced. The word is beautiful, and very often deceiving. I do not recommend it to you. However, I advise you to give life by teaching the infinite or the Order of the Universe. And this, not with words, but in deeds.

"To accept everything and to give everything" is a yardstick that will reveal to you your own state of illness or of health. Turn yourself into one who has supreme judging ability, absolute justice, infinite freedom, and eternal happiness.

THE FAITH THAT MOVES MOUNTAINS

If you have faith, nothing shall be impossible to you. Crimes, hostility, poverty, wars, and especially so-called incurable illness are all the end result of a lack of faith.

Happiness or unhappiness depends upon our behavior, which, in turn, is controlled by our judgment. Faith is the solid foundation upon which judgment rises.

We must not confuse that type of judgment that is based on faith with the variety that is not. The judgment that fails is the latter. If your judgment fails, you are one who has not even as much faith as a grain of mustard seed. Faith is judgment in infinity. If you do not know the Order of the Universe, you have no faith. If you have confidence only in manmade contrivances such as laws, power, knowledge, science, money, drugs, and medicines, you have faith only in relativity, not in infinity. Since all relative judgment is transitory and of little value, you should learn the structure of infinity: the eternal creator.

This is why I have spent so many years as an interpreter of the philosophy of the ancient Far East and why I have designed this guidebook. It is a passport to the kingdom of health, freedom, and happiness, where every being is his own master, free and healthy, never salaried, never dependent. Birds, fish, insects, and microbes along with all herbs and trees live there in

Message From Lima Ohsawa

Reprinted from *The Macrobiotic*, May 1966

Dear Macrobiotic friends all over the world,

What sad, sudden news I must give you.

The founder of the macrobiotic movement and beloved teacher of the philosophy of the Far East, Mr. George Ohsawa, died on April 24, at 5:30 P.M. Although I was with him at the time of his sudden passing, I am at a loss to offer a complete explanation for this shocking occurrence. I must apologize.

*Mr. Ohsawa arose on the morning of April 24th at the usual hour of 3 A.M. and finished editing his Japanese magazine as well as a pamphlet concerning our summer camp, *The Cultural and Spiritual Olympics*.*

At twelve noon, we both attended the meeting of a new macrobiotic organization where he spoke for one hour. After returning home in the rain at three, he sat at his desk re-reading his article for the next issue of the magazine. This was typical of our daily routine. A while later, I said, "It is time for dinner." We were alone. As he started the meal, Mr. Ohsawa remarked, "Today is very quiet . . . we haven't had that in a long time, don't you think?"

After two or three mouthsful of food, he stood up suddenly. I rushed to his side in alarm. As I reached him, he fell on my arm with a groan. I checked his pulse, but I could feel none on either wrist. I palm-treated his heart and massaged his back . . . he groaned again. "Be strong," I cried.

I was encouraged to see that he drank a cup of shoban (bancha tea and soy sauce) that I prepared, but still I could not find his pulse.

"Can you recognize me?" He nodded.

"You must not die." Again he nodded.

"Shall I call Dr. Ushio?" He refused my offer . . . he wanted me to cure him. At this time, our friend Mr. Okawa appeared and I asked him to help.

"Where is the pain?"

"In the back," was the faint reply.

Mr. Okawa and I nursed him and prayed but the pain continued. I sensed that there was something final about the situation and decided to call the doctor. When I returned to Mr. Ohsawa's side after calling Drs. Ushio and Takase, he inhaled twice and became very still. His eyes remained open.

"Oh no!" I couldn't believe that he had died so I resumed massaging him. Drs. Ushio and Takase arrived soon after. They tried heart massage, artificial respiration, and other treatment to no avail . . . it was too late . . . there was no way to save him. The four of us just sat and said nothing. Only two or three minutes had elapsed from the time that his last pain began until he expired, but it had seemed like hours. I cried out but there was no reply. Could it really be that George Ohsawa was gone? I lost all my energy and fell to the floor crying.

Why had this happened? His heart had stopped instantly as if something had speared it.

Perhaps the answer lies in an examination of his activities shortly before death. He had been trying to make a macrobiotic drink from Chinese herbs for three or four months. Every morning, he mixed up a new test brew, tasted it, and offered some to me. Sometimes it was bitter, at other times sour. I asked him to stop these experiments many times, but he was a man who never gave up until he achieved success. "I will make a drink with the taste of malt liquor." In addition, he had recently begun to use beni-hana (rouge flower) because it had been said that this secret herb would aid cancer victims. Not long ago, he had gotten a headache which I dissipated by palm treatment. This happened more than once and each time, I was able to rid him of the pain.

Some of his hair fell out and the scalp became itchy. Small bumps appeared at the back of his head just a few days ago. They disappeared after I treated them with my palm. This may have been traces of the filaria (blood parasites) from which he suffered about ten years ago in Africa. Only this morning (April 24th), mucous came out of his head.

Filaria may have attacked his heart. Or, he might have been overworked beyond human endurance. He only slept two or three hours a day and spent the rest of the time writing, editing, answering the many letters that came to him from all over the world, attending various meetings and conferences, and helping to organize the macrobiotic movement throughout the world. Such living must have taken its toll. The cause of his death has been diagnosed as arterial thrombosis by four Japanese doctors who are macrobiotic.

This announcement of the untimely death of my husband, Mr. George Ohsawa, is made with deep sadness and regret.

He has passed away but his teaching will remain within us forever.

Mrs. Lima Ohsawa

Editorial by Lou Oles following Lima's message:

It is with deep sorrow that the Ohsawa Foundation has published Mrs. Lima Ohsawa's letter. With the passing of George Ohsawa, we have lost a friend, a father, a true teacher, a benevolent task-master . . . but above all, we have lost the most positive influence that we have known in our lives.

An over-wrought friend has asked, "What ever will you do now that your god is dead?"

What a total lack of understanding. George Ohsawa was not a god to the people who knew him either through his work or through personal contact. It is enough that he was a vibrant, happy, active, and inspiring human being. How fortunate for us to have crossed his path.

His first lectures in New York City are a vivid memory. There, Mr. Ohsawa defined the happy man as one who:

thinks . . .
has faith . . .
has a billion friends . . .
knows freedom . . .
can change men . . .
knows God . . .
is an adventurer . . .

That night in September of 1960, he was sketching his self-portrait:

he was a thinker of the most profound order . . .
he had an abiding faith in the Order of the Universe . . .
his friends, East and West, are without number . . .
he knew the freedom of detachment from the petty, material
    world that enabled him to "give, give, and give" endlessly
    of himself so that our understanding might be unveiled . . .
both his presence and words have changed the lives of millions
    and will continue to do so long after we are gone . . .
that he knew God is apparent if we examine the work that was
    his life . . .
the details of his passing bear final witness to the fact that he
    was above all the greatest adventurer, always striving to
    deepen his understanding of life. He died in the way he
    taught us to live: "The bigger the difficulty, the bigger the
    pleasure." . . .

We, who are left behind, face the future with the humility, the
smiling faces, the sense of responsibility, and the deep purpose that
would have made Ohsawa the happiest of men.

complete satisfaction without knowing the fear of sickness, old age, or death. I shall be very happy if you can use this passport even for only ten days. If you decide to be happy, free, healthy, and independent through observing the directions of my philosophy, contact me anytime and anywhere via the telephone called faith.

Faith means the spiritual quality of a small and very happy child. It is the state of mind of the kingdom of heaven, which knows nothing of human laws or morals.

Faith, the supreme integral wisdom, has a quality that is totally transparent, with the power to permeate all things. In outward appearance it is elegant, graceful, and full of joy. Thus, true faith is not credo or belief, it is complete wisdom or understanding of truth. In essence, it is justice or freedom; in appearance, it is love and joy. Let me explain it in a parable: Faith is an ocean of wisdom with neither surface nor floor, without end in either space or time, and yet all is in perfect order. There is not one infinitesimal particle, even of infinite speed, that is working outside of this universal solidarity. Because of its great speed and the ultra-transparency of its constitution, nothing can be detected by sight or sense in this ocean but elegantly dancing myriads of pearls like bubbles of joy, moving spirally in all directions.

The traditional faith of the Far East is a resonance produced in the individual (small self) by the greatest individuality (large self, the infinite universe); it is not an illusory connection or a fleeting communication between one individual and another.

Many people, curiously enough, believe that the seat of thought, imagination, and the mind encompassed by our memory is found in the brain. Actually, this is somewhat reversed. Our body, especially the brain, is an instrument like a radio receiver that automatically picks up any frequency. This automatic quality itself is that which is known as memory, thought, and imagination. Thus, our small brain is like a connection to the large "brain" of the universe itself. These things, as well as the powers of reasoning and will, are not merely a receiver that picks up radio waves; they are like a very advanced and sensitive television set that operates in time—in the past, the present, and the future. Within our brain alone, there are at least ten billion vacuum tubes called cells. Our body is soaked in the depths of the infinite undulating ocean of the pre-electronic waves of mind, soul, or spirit. Our thinking mind is not contained within this fragile and ephemeral prison of the body; quite the contrary. For this very reason we are able to think, imagine, memorize, and compare one scene with another.

Our body is immersed to the marrow of our bones in the ocean of super-high-speed electronic waves over the Earth that are constantly passing through us. The speed of the Earth's rotation around the sun plus the speed of the sun also moving around the Milky Way galaxy, combined with the movement of our Earth as it also spins on its own axis while receiving this influence, equals a tremendous speed. Every instant, every second, our actions here on this Earth are projected at this ultra-super speed into the far reaches of space. It is like a scene from a movie. At first, it is all rolled up and put away within the film case, but when it becomes extended through the lens of the miraculous extrasensory projector of our mind and realized on the screen of our consciousness, we are able to witness all the variety of life's scenes every moment and from any place. This is certainly the most complicated of all projectors.

Faith, like that of Jesus, is the strength and the mechanism behind such a mind. This miraculous projector projects scenes one after another in front of its lens at a tremendous speed. Furthermore, it is able to select and magnify any part of any scene, even one that has already been rolled up and put away, completely at its own discretion. Indeed, it is the multi-origin projector of all scenes. At the same time, it is also the light that illuminates them whenever we want to view them. It is the film, the playwright, the set designer, the scene painter, the orchestra, the conductor, the cameraman, the producer, the actors, and even the paying spectators. It writes, produces, and projects as it wishes. The mind is the one infinite ocean of life, while physical bodies are infinitely numerous.

Physical bodies appear and fade away again like the foam on the ocean tide. But their Creator brings them forth and distinguishes them one from the other, and this allows us to establish understanding among ourselves. It is also the very reason why we tend to personify all other existences as well and treat them as if they were human. Such an attitude is not total ignorance. It is not blind faith or the attitude of a beggar who, with tears in his eyes, pleads for the grace of the Divine Creator. God is also unnecessary. We are ephemeral and illusory foam, physiologically speaking, but at the same time—because we have mind and feeling—we are also the creator of that infinite ocean of mind. Each of us contains this two-sided dialectic constitution. Therefore, even within the same individual there is a constant conflict of body and soul (heart and mind), and this of course is prevalent among the greater majority of people.

Jesus cured everything by faith, which is nothing else than everlasting prayer. But everlasting prayer or faith must not be confused with supplication. It is the permanent awareness and the penetrating contemplation of the principles of the universe; the infinite, omnipresent, omnipotent, and omniscient. Faith, according to all the great religions of the Far East, including Christianity, is not a creed (*credo quia absurdum*) but a clearsighted understanding of the Order of the Universe, through all the finite, transient, and illusory phenomena, internally; externally, it is the love that embraces everything without exclusiveness and with eternal joyfulness.

We are greedy, we always eat in excess; that is why fasting (eating and drinking simply) is the only door, open to all, through which we can view and enjoy the splendid panorama of the world of faith. The poorer one is, the nearer one is to that door, since there is always some hunger in *vivere parvo*, living simply and naturally.

The following is an interpretation of the law of contradiction. The first two principles of the seven logical principles of the Unifying Principle (see page 121) are:

1. Whatever has a beginning has an end.
2. That which has a front has a back.

These are the backbone of all the great religions; they must be substituted for the formal Kantian logic, which is the foundation of modern Western science and philosophy and the origin of the evils that exist today. They, and they only, translate this mutation and explain its mechanism.

Beginning is opposite and antagonistic to ending. In this relative, material world, the front is antithetical and opposed to the back. In the end, happiness leads to sadness, life to death, beauty to ugliness, activity to weariness, strength to weakness. Everything comes to an end, which is the opposite of its beginning; everything is supported, animated, maintained, and destroyed by its opposite. This is the great law of nature, which I call the Order of the Universe. It is the very mysterious and great law that rules our life in this relative world (but not in the absolute, eternal, and infinite one).

If this is understood, there will be no more difficulty in curing so-called incurable illnesses. Without knowing or understanding this great concept of the universe, fundamental cure will be impossible.

In Africa, I once saw a clergyman, aged sixty-two. He had spent a quiet pious life, devoted to God. After a long life of duties, he was plagued by many misfortunes: cataract (one eye out of use), prostate inflammation, heart illness, chronic ulcers at the feet that did not heal (perhaps of leprous origin), urodynia, etc. Why did God send these diseases to this pious clergyman? For over fifteen years his wife had suffered queer troubles: ceaseless headaches, pricking pains shifting through her whole body, continuous blinking, inflammation of the lachrymal ducts, and gum pains, notwithstanding the fact that she had lost most of her teeth. In addition, she had been operated on twice for ovarian troubles, and after that, her abdomen had ached constantly.

After so long a life devoted to God, at the age of sixty-two, does one still have to suffer? Is that life? What is the sense of a pious Christian life? He never had real faith, but for over forty years he had believed deeply in God's mercy. Where is the heavenly kingdom? Where is God? Were his many years of preaching a deception? He had exhausted his strength.

Happiness as the barometer or yardstick of one's life depends on our supreme judging ability. He who possesses clearsightedness is endowed with the vision not only of all that exists in this relative world, but also in the infinite (the past as well as the future), and will never be unhappy. This is real faith. But this man did not possess this kind of faith. What he held to and believed to be faith was a blind creed, a poor slave's principle. It was a baseless trust, blind ignorance, though a very brave one (*credo quia absurdum*, the belief in something sheerly because it is so incredible). This ignorance they call "faith" is a false passport that is delivered by religious professionals.

The clergyman and his wife had clearly realized that there was no medication or operation that could heal them. But, still being dependent on medicine, they did not understand Jesus's faith. Faith is total independence, infinite freedom, eternal happiness, and absolute justice. Once this faith is well established, there will be nothing impossible for you; you will suffer no more pain, and with still more reason, have no fear. You will never again depend upon anyone or upon any instrument.

The clergyman and his wife showed nothing but yin symptoms, primarily those of too much sugar. Being a churchman, he had more opportunities to get chocolates, cakes, sugar, and fruit than others in the community. They quite clearly understood me and promised to purify themselves from their "original sin," from the crimes they had committed against the physiological and biological laws of life's creation, i.e., the selection, assortment, and preparation of their foods, and the way to eat them. To eat is to create a new life for tomorrow through the sacrifice of the vegetal realm and its products. If mistakes are made, this is, literally, the "original sin." This is symbolized in the myth of the Garden of Eden.

I was, however, greatly inspired by the clergyman. Even a humble African, a pious servant for the whole of his innocent and primitive life, could understand that palliative and symptomatic medicine ought to be replaced by faith; and also, that faith is the other name for the supreme omnipotent medicine that cures every physiological, psychological, or spiritual illness. Trying to cure disease by prickings or medications is the product of a low, eclipsed, and veiled judging ability.

What is the relationship between medicine and faith: Is it magic? Or superstition? A great many authors, especially religious ones, assert that disease can be cured by faith. Dr. Alexis Carrel, author of that revealing volume *Man, the Unknown* was wholly convinced that, among the believers in the Lourdes miracles, there were miraculous recoveries.

Modern medicine does not deny that there are in the structures and functions of the human body many marvels; medicine cannot account for them no matter how developed physicians and the medicine they practice may seem. These marvels cannot be explained. Those who have faith, those who insist upon its importance and superiority cannot, themselves, explain its processes. But he who does not know his plane's mechanism cannot be a good pilot and may not be trusted. How much more important it is for physicians to know life in all its manifestations—the body and mind in all their expressions.

To believe in modern symptomatic medicine and its techniques is superstition; it is a slave's mentality, and such belief or confidence leads very often to tragedy. Such faith has no reason; it is mere sentimentality and it is synonymous with ignorance. The faith that heals only symptoms is sentimental and not real.

If, on the contrary, medicine is provided with a universal compass (the Order of the Universe or the Unifying Principle) that shows correct orientation, it is likely to progress in the right direction a thousandfold in the next twenty-five years. Medical studies simply must begin with an understanding of the constitution of life and the universe.

Strangely enough, many of those who preach the "power of faith" and the miraculous healings of Jesus and also of the great Buddhists swallow medicaments they buy in drugstores and go to hospitals to be cured by empiric and symptomatic medicine. Why, then, do they preach the importance and superiority of faith? All that they preach about faith is true and exact, but they do not know what faith is. They are but phonographs. They have to learn first by study and experience that faith is the perfect understanding and realization of the Order of the Universe and its Unifying Principle (in old-fashioned terminology: the kingdom of heaven and its justice).

According to the Unifying Principle, the greatest thing in life is faith. Internally, this faith is a clairvoyance (opposite to that of *credo quia absurdum est*) that clearly sees and comprehends everything through infinite time and space. Externally, it is a manifestation of universal love or supreme judgment, embracing all antagonisms and transforming them into oneness, distributing the eternal joy of life to all, forever. It is the kind of faith that sends the mountain into the sea and that insures infinite freedom, eternal happiness, and absolute justice.

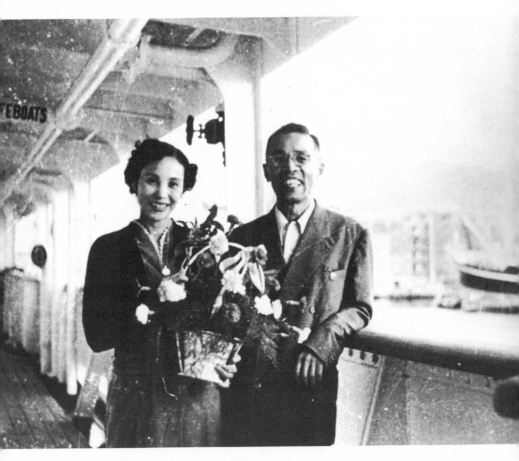

George Ohsawa departs Japan on his way to India with his wife, Lima, October 1953.

END NOTE

George Ohsawa believed beyond the shadow of a doubt that he had found, and was teaching to others, the key to the kingdom of heaven—a practical way to understand the Order of the Universe and one's place in that order. In the face of such incredible truth, all problems such as pain, suffering, anxiety, fear, and sickness melt into their opposites and a life with real joy results.

In this age of fifteen-second sound bites, push-button information, and fast-acting medications, it has become natural for people to want answers in outline form. They expect the very key to happiness in an easy-to-understand condensed version in the preface and introduction so that they needn't read the whole book. This is simply not possible. The key is simple enough but clouded thinking and judging ability get in the way of understanding it. To clear this cloudiness takes years of discipline and practice in eating and drinking a simple, natural diet. My own experience is an example.

When I attended my first French Meadows macrobiotic summer camp more than fifteen years ago, I was impressed by the vitality and clarity of the people who had been practicing macrobiotics more than ten years. They walked without stiffness, viewed nature with deep appreciation in their eyes, and radiated a real sense of joy in living. Now, I, too, know the joy of less cloudy thinking.

Many people have begun macrobiotic practice since Ohsawa first began teaching. Many have continued, some have stopped;

some have found the key, others haven't. Actually there are many keys and many doors, and you must find the right key for you in order to open the door of your choice. The first step is to read this book and begin natural eating and drinking. Then, reread this book often to see how your understanding deepens as your practice continues.

There are many macrobiotic centers that can help and support you in your search. Two of the largest in the United States are the George Ohsawa Macrobiotic Foundation, PO Box 3998, Chico, CA 95927-3998; (800) 232-2372, fax (530) 566-9768 and the Kushi Institute, Box 7 Leland Road, Becket, MA 01223; (413) 623-5742, fax (413) 827-8827. Either center can help you, put you in touch with a local contact, or provide a list of macrobiotic books and/or suppliers.

As you embark upon macrobiotic practice, you would do well to remember George Ohsawa's words in *Magic Spectacles,* a play written for children.

No precisely-produced camera can compare with your eye.
No airplane, jet, or atomic-powered engine can compare with
    your heart.
No great building can compare with your body cells.

The most important thing to do is to clear up the clouds in
    your thinking or judging ability.
This is the aim or goal of my teaching.

The world is big.
You are young.
There are many places to go; there are many things to do.
The only thing you need is health.

If you know the secret of health and observe it, then you will
    gain freedom and independence.
How wonderful life is if you apply this principle of life by
    yourself.
Life becomes more interesting than the adventures of Tom
    Sawyer.

You can do anything you want to do all of your life.
What a great life lies before you!

CHRONOLOGY
OF GEORGE
OHSAWA'S LIFE

1893 George Ohsawa is born to Magotaro and Setsuko Sakurazawa, both of the samurai class, on October 18 near the Kennin-ti Temple in Kyoto, Japan, and named Yukikazu Sakurazawa.

1899 His father divorces Setsuko and leaves her, Ohsawa, and a youger brother to fend for themselves. Ohsawa and his brother often go without socks, shoes, and overcoats, even in the wintertime.

1903 His mother contracts pulmonary tuberculosis when Ohsawa is nine and dies after months of illness. Ohsawa begins to take care of his younger brother. A younger sister had already died in infancy.

1908 He develops tuberculosis of the lungs and intestines, and other sicknesses.

1911 When Ohsawa is eighteen, his brother dies of tuberculosis and Ohsawa's tuberculosis and other conditions worsen. Doctors give him little chance of survival.

1912 Ohsawa re-establishes his health using Sagen Ishizuka's diet of whole brown rice, fresh vegetables, sea salt, and oil.

1913 He graduates from commercial high school, moves to the international port city of Kobe, and begins studying French. He had already begun to learn English and had a great interest in both Japanese and Western literature.

1914 Ohsawa is employed by England's Wormth Steamship Company as a ship's purser and, during World War I, travels to Europe for the first time. Along the way, he is exposed to Southeast Asia, India, and Egypt, fulfilling his desire to see the world outside Japan.

1915 He is employed by Nakagiri Trading Company in Kobe as a manager.

1916 He joins Shoku-Yo Kai, an organization carrying on the work of Sagen Ishizuka whose regime had saved his life a few years earlier. He begins to distribute food, organize meetings and lectures, and contribute articles to the organization's monthly magazine.

1917 Ohsawa becomes a manager of the Kobe branch of the Kumasawa Trading Company, whose main business is in textiles, and begins to travel to Europe every other year.

1919 He starts a movement for Japanese language reform through the publication of a magazine called *Rebirth*.

1920 He brings the first broadcast radio transmitter and receiver from France to Japan and invents a device that improves existing movie and still cameras. His translation of Charles Baudelaire's *Les Fleurs du Mal (The Flowers of Evil)* is published in Japanese. In these ways, Ohsawa begins to introduce Western culture to the Japanese, a role that will continue throughout his life. At the same time, he continues to study the classics of Far Eastern traditions.

1923 An earthquake and fire in Tokyo destroy his company's home office. Control of the company is taken over by the investors and he decides to quit the business.

1924 Ohsawa moves to Tokyo and begins his life work by rejoining the Shoku-Yo Kai movement full-time.

1927 He becomes a supervisor of Shoku-Yo Kai and is named editor of the magazine *Shokuyo*, which in essence means "macrobiotic." His writings begin to emphasize Japanese spirit and culture instead of Western culture, and he publishes *The Physiology of the Japanese Spirit*, a collection of magazine articles.

1928 Ohsawa holds the first macrobiotic summer camp in Hokkaido and publishes a biography of Sagen Ishizuka and five volumes of *The Shoku-Yo Seminars: Discourse on Macrobiotics*. He criticizes Western culture, especially its science and medicine, and praises the medicine of the Far East.

1929 At age thirty-five, he resigns from Shoku-Yo Kai, where he is a leading figure, makes arrangements for the care of his dependents from second and third marriages that had each ended in divorce, and leaves Japan to live in France and to teach (spread) the Shoku-Yo philosophy to the West. Without any financial support, he visits Paris via the Trans-Siberian railway—a fourteen-day trip on cushionless benches with brown rice as his only food.

1930 Although living a very poor life in Paris, he manages to study at both the Sorbonne University and the Pasteur Institute at the age of thirty-seven. At the same time, he teaches Far Eastern medicine, acupuncture, flower arrangement, judo, and haiku to the French people.

1931 Ohsawa publishes *The Unique Principle*, in which he tries to explain the world view and culture of the Far East to the Western people, and *The Book of Flowers* in French under the name Georges Ohsawa. He begins to meet some of the writers whose works he had been studying. However, he is largely unsuccessful at convincing them of his ideas.

1932 He returns to Japan to try to convince the new Japanese nationalists and militarists that their foreign policies will eventually lead to a disastrous confrontation with Western powers. He publishes *Why Japan Must Fight With the White Race*, in which he pleads for peace by trying to clear up misunderstandings and by exchanging ideologies. The subtitle, *No Reason*, is virtually ignored and the book doesn't produce the hoped-for change. Ohsawa returns to France after a few months.

1935 He returns again to his native Japan to help change the direction of those in charge away from war and ultimate disaster. He immediately begins lecturing and writing and becomes active once again in the Shoku-Yo Kai. He will soon become editor-in-chief of publications and general superintendent.

1936 He publishes several books on diet and medicine and meets his future wife, Sanae Tanaka.

1937 He asks Sanae to join his household. She agrees and they live as a common-law couple before being married ten years later. Ohsawa renames her Lima and she frees him from household tasks so that he can devote even more time to writing, lecturing, and travelling. He begins publishing yet another magazine called *Musubi*, meaning "to bring together." He also publishes *Who Are Those Who Destroy Japan?*, which provokes strong reaction from military leaders. Out of self-protection, he becomes health consultant to the Emperor's family and other nobles.

1938 The subscribers to the magazine *Shokuyo* reach ten thousand. He translates and publishes Alexis Carrel's *Man the Unknown* in Japanese and writes a four-hundred-page book entitled *Nature Medicine* in just five days. Many of his books during this time are hastily written because of the urgency he feels in affecting a change in people's ways. He visits Manchuria in September, giving lectures and consultations, and publishes several reports of his ideas to improve their conditions.

1939   Ohsawa publishes *A New Dietetic Cure,* which sells millions of copies in Japanese. He resigns from the Shoku-Yo Kai and continues his warnings of the inadvisability of war.

1940   He founds the Unique Principle Lecture and Research Center in Ohtsu City, where he teaches yin-yang theory instead of how to symptomatically cure diseases. He begins organizing and conducting summer camps for children and a summer school for adults. Being very interested in the education of children, he writes *The Magic Spectacles,* a play for children to perform that teaches them the importance of food and yin-yang theory. On September 5th, he and three helpers are arrested for violation of medical law, treated very roughly in jail, and then released due to a lack of evidence. He is not intimidated and continues his activities.

1941   Ohsawa issues ten thousand copies of *Standing on the Front Line of the Health War,* once again provoking military leaders. He warns them that they will destroy Japan and bring confusion to the country similar to that during the French Revolution. He also predicts that they will be shot. His prophecy will be realized four years later at the end of the war. However, his warning is so strong that there is grave danger of his assassination. The Japanese Government bans *Who Are Those Who Destroy Japan?* and two thousand copies are burned. Ohsawa is detained several times for interrogation. He begins work on a forty-eight-volume set of writings on the Unifying Principle with the publication of two books, *The Order of the Universe* and *The Order of Man.* He will complete over half of this massive project.

1942   He publishes *The New Science of Nutrition, The Phenomena of Life and the Environment,* and *A New Study of the Seven Articles on Military Strategy.* He begins to despair of politics because no one will listen to him. Pressure from the military government increases.

1943 Ohsawa publishes *The Last and Eternal Winner* in which he predicts that England will free India and that Gandhi will be killed. This prophecy comes true a couple of years later. He also publishes *Primitive Mentality and the Japanese Mentality*, which he had promised to write for René Levy-Bruhl more than ten years earlier.

1944 He again predicts that Japan will be defeated. To all students at the front he sends telegrams reading: "You should be careful in eating and be the last winner," meaning that it is more important to survive than to follow orders. He publishes two more anti-war and anti-militaristic books: *Eternal Children: Anatole France and Romain Rolland*, admiring the French idealistic pacifists, and *How to Cure the Heart*, explaining how to end militarism by natural living. In November, he tries to reach Moscow through Manchuria in order to ask Russia to mediate between Japan and the Western powers. En route, he is chased by the military police and forced to change his plan. He escapes capture, however, and returns to Japan to plan another attempt.

1945 In January, he is captured in his hide-out and jailed under very severe conditions, the temperature often going to five degrees below zero. He is forced to undergo frequent torturous interrogation. After three months in jail, he loses 80 percent of his vision and almost dies. He survives due to foods sent by Lima and others. At the end of June, he is suddenly released with the stipulation that he will not bring a law suit against the government. In July, he attempts a coup aided by Generals Imura and Ujimori, but he is captured again, sent to prison, and sentenced to death. In August, Japan surrenders and in September, Ohsawa is released by order of General MacArthur just before execution of the death sentence. In October, he publishes *Why Was Japan Defeated?* in which he outlines his vision for Japan's future based on a return to natural eating and living. In December, he founds The True Way of Life Cooperative Center, a new educational center, in Tokyo.

1946 Ohsawa founds two other educational centers in Yokohama. He begins publication of the monthly magazine *Compas*.

1947 He moves to the Myorenji district of Yokohama and establishes the Maison Ignoramus (House of the Ignorant). He joins the United World Federalists Organization to broaden the scope of his activities. He adopts the name "macrobiotics" to describe his all-encompassing view of life and changes his name from Yukikazu Sakurazawa to George Ohsawa. Ohsawa is a reading of Sakurazawa using a mid-1800s Chinese pronunciation. A similar reading of his first name yields Nyoichi, a name that is often used in reference to him.

1948 He moves his Maison Ignoramus to the Hiyoshi district of Yokohama and changes the name to The World Government Center. The government bars him from holding public office because of his writings during the war. He begins publication of another magazine called *Health,* and a newspaper called *World Government,* which is published every ten days. He sends his suggestions for solving the world's problems to more than one hundred prominent people and receives only one reply, an invitation from Dr. Albert Schweitzer in Africa to come visit. This he will do several years later.

1949 Ohsawa is active in the world government movement in various cities, basing his approach on the idea that world peace is only possible when individuals first establish their own health and happiness through biological and physiological improvement, that is, eating the proper foods. He meets Norman Cousins at a World Federalist conference in Hiroshima. At his World Government Center, he begins training people to send around the world as macrobiotic missionaries.

1950 He returns to his respect for Western cultures and traditions and again focuses on uniting East and West. He begins to read and study American and British writings, producing a period of intellectual and personal growth. He translates and publishes F.S.C. Northrop's *The Meeting of East and West* in two volumes in Japanese, calling it one of the most significant books of the twentieth century, and corresponds with Northrop.

1952 He publishes *The Eternal Youth: Biography of Benjamin Franklin* in Japanese and *The Book of Judo* in French.

1953 He writes *Gandhi, the Eternal Youth*. The travel ban against him is lifted and so at age sixty, Ohsawa, accompanied by Lima, leaves Japan for India to teach macrobiotics to the world.

1954 He reads the classics of Indian literature and founds the Indo-Japan Cultural Center in India. In an open letter to Mao Tse-Tung, he advises him on his health and on Chinese policies from the standpoint of macrobiotic thinking. Despite Ohsawa's continual letters to his students back in Japan, the World Government Center starts to break apart and diminishes in its ability to promote the activities Ohsawa had begun.

1955 Ohsawa leaves India by boat for Africa to meet Dr. Albert Schweitzer. He arrives in Lambarené in the Belgian Congo and begins teaching macrobiotics to the Africans. He purposely contracts tropical ulcers, thought to be a fatal disease, and cures himself in ten days using a macrobiotic diet. He advises Dr. Schweitzer to adopt the macrobiotic approach for his patients, but Schweitzer disagrees. Ohsawa leaves Lambarené and goes to Paris, where twenty-five years previously, he had planted the seeds of Far Eastern culture.

1956 He lectures day and night on macrobiotics in Belgium, Switzerland, Germany, Sweden, Italy, and England. A macrobiotic foods factory (LIMA) opens in Belgium, and macrobiotic stores and restaurants open all over Europe. *The Philosophy of Oriental Medicine*, Ohsawa's book to explain macrobiotic thinking to Dr. Schweitzer and the West, is published in French.

1957 He begins publishing the monthly French magazine *Yin Yang*.

1958 Ohsawa writes *Jack and Mitie in the West* in French, showing his disappointment in the French (Western) people's low level of comprehension of the spirit of Far Eastern culture.

1959 At the age of sixty-six, Ohsawa visits the United States for the first time.

1960 He publishes *Zen Macrobiotics* in mimeograph form in New York. The first American macrobiotic magazine, *Macrobiotic News*, is started in January in New York. He gives ten-day seminars during January, February, and March. He returns to Europe in April and goes back to the United States in July, lecturing every weekend for two months at the first American macrobiotic summer camp on Long Island.

1961 He leads the second American Summer Camp in Wurtzboro, New York, in July and August with great success. On the advice of Ohsawa, thirteen macrobiotic families (thirty-seven people in all) leave New York in a car caravan and move to Chico, California, to avoid possible nuclear fallout from an attack by the Soviet Union.

1962 Ohsawa holds another successful summer camp in France. The first American macrobiotic food manufacturing and distributing company (Chico San) is established in Chico by those families Ohsawa had advised to move to California. He publishes *The Atomic Age and the Philosophy of the Far East* in French.

1963 He lectures in New York and Boston, and at the Chico summer camp. His prediction that President Kennedy may be assassinated draws media attention. This prediction will be realized later in the year.

1964 In Japan, he and his disciples succeed in an experiment in atomic transmutation on July 21st. Shortly afterward, he lectures in California at the Big Sur Summer Camp. He publishes *Cancer and the Philosophy of the Far East*, his last major book, in French.

1965 Ohsawa commences to organize a Spiritual Olympics in Japan. His idea is to bring together one hundred visitors from the West and one hundred Japanese people in order to promote mutual understanding and cooperation. *You Are All Sanpaku*, a reworking of Ohsawa's texts by writer William Dufty, is published in English. Ohsawa continues to lecture throughout Europe and the United States.

1966 Ohsawa writes "Educating the Will" and at age seventy-two, he dies suddenly on April 24th of what is diagnosed as a heart attack. Followers continue to publish works based on his theories and lectures along with new translations and editions of his voluminous writings. The Spiritual Olympics originated by him is held in Japan in July and August and is attended by over one hundred macrobiotic people from all over the world.

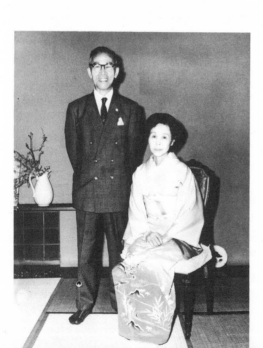

April-17-1966-
photo of George Ohsawa
taken one week
before his death.

THE WRITINGS OF GEORGE OHSAWA

ENGLISH TITLES

Acupuncture and the Philosophy of the Far East. Tao Books, Boston, 1973. Originally published as *L'Acupuncture et la Médecine d'Extrême Orient,* Librarie J. Vrin, Paris, 1934. Out of print.

The Art of Peace. George Ohsawa Macrobiotic Foundation, Oroville, California, 1990. Originally published as *Le Livre du Judo: Commetaire sur le Principes des Écoles de "Do" (The Book of Judo: Commentary on the Principles of the Schools of the Way)* by Centre Ignoramus de Paris, Paris, 1952.

Atomic Age and the Philosophy of the Far East. George Ohsawa Macrobiotic Foundation, Oroville, California, 1977. Originally published as *L'Ere Atomique et la Philosophie d'Extrême Orient* by Librarie J. Vrin, Paris, 1962. Out of print.

Biological Transmutations: Natural Alchemy, with Louis Kervran. George Ohsawa Macrobiotic Foundation, Oroville, California, 1976. First edition, 1971. Originally published as *Biological Atomic Transmutation,* with Louis Kervran, in Japan in 1962. Out of print.

The Book of Flowers. See *Le Livre des Fleurs* in Original French Titles.

The Book of Judo. See *The Art of Peace* above.

The Book of Judgment. See *The Philosophy of Oriental Medicine* on page 225.

But I Love Fruits, with Neven Henaff and Jacques de Langre. Pamphlet. Happiness Press, Magalia, California, undated. Originally published in English as *Vitamin C and Fruit* by George Ohsawa Macrobiotic Foundation, 1971. Ohsawa's part was taken from an article written in English in the early 1960s.

Cancer and the Philosophy of the Far East. See *Macrobiotics: The Way of Healing,* above.

Four Hours to Basic Japanese. George Ohsawa Macrobiotic Foundation, Oroville, California, 1973. Originally written in English in the early 1960s. Out of print.

Gandhi: The Eternal Youth. George Ohsawa Macrobiotic Foundation, Oroville, California, 1990. Originally published as *Eien no Shonen—Tsuzuki: Gandhi no Shonen Jidai (The Eternal Youth—Continued: Gandhi's Youth)* in Japan, 1954.

Jack and Mitie in the West. George Ohsawa Macrobiotic Foundation, Oroville, California, 1981. Originally published as *Jack et Madame Mitie en Occident* by Librarie J. Vrin, Paris, 1958. Out of print.

Jack and Yoyo in Erewhon. A comic book published in Japanese and English by Sekai Seihu Kyokai, Japan, date unavailable. Out of print.

Life and Death. George Ohsawa Macrobiotic Foundation, Oroville, California, 1984. Pamphlet. Originally written in English in the early 1960s.

Macrobiotic Guidebook for Living. George Ohsawa Macrobiotic Foundation, Oroville, California, 1985. Originally published as *Shoku-yo Jinsei Tokuhon: Hito no Issho no Sekkei (The Shoku-Yo Guidebook for Living: A Plan for a Human Lifetime)* in Japan, 1938. First major English edition was *Macrobiotic Guidebook for Living: The Philosophy of Oriental Medicine, Volume 3* by The Ohsawa Foundation, Los Angeles, 1966.

Macrobiotics: An Invitation to Health and Happiness, with Herman

Aihara. George Ohsawa Macrobiotic Foundation, Oroville, California, 1971. Ohsawa's part was originally published as *An Invitation to Health and Happiness* in Japan in 1965.

Macrobiotics: The Way of Healing. George Ohsawa Macrobiotic Foundation, Oroville, California, 1984. Originally published as *Le Cancer et la Philosophie d'Extrême Orient (Cancer and the Philosophy of the Far East)* by Librarie J. Vrin, Paris, 1964. First published in English as *Cancer and the Philosophy of the Far East* by Swan House in 1971.

The Order of the Universe. George Ohsawa Macrobiotic Foundation, Oroville, California, 1986. Originally published as *Uchu no Chitsujo (The Order of the Universe)* in Japan, 1941. UP I:1.*

Philosophy of Oriental Medicine. George Ohsawa Macrobiotic Foundation, Oroville, California, 1991. Originally published as *Le Philosophie de la Médecine d'Extrême Orient* by Librarie J. Vrin, Paris, 1956, and as *Toyo Igaku no Tetsugaku (The Philosophy of Oriental Medicine)* in Japan, 1958. First major English edition was *The Book of Judgment: The Philosophy of Oriental Medicine, Volume 2* by the Ohsawa Foundation, Los Angeles, 1966.

Practical Guide to Far Eastern Macrobiotic Medicine. George Ohsawa Macrobiotic Foundation, Oroville, California, 1973. The idea for this book came from *Guide Pratique de la Médecine d'Extrême Orient* published by Chez L'Auteur in Paris in 1956. Actually the book is a translation of many of Ohsawa's writings compiled and edited by Herman Aihara. Out of print.

Smoking, Marijuana and Drugs, with Herman Aihara and Fred Pulver. George Ohsawa Macrobiotic Foundation, Oroville, California, 1984. Pamphlet. Originally written in English in the early 1960s.

Two Great Indians in Japan: Sri Rash Behari Bose and Netaji Subhas Chandra Bose. Indo-Japanese Cultural Association, Calcutta, 1954. Out of print.

---

* *UPI:1 stands for Unique Principle Series Volume 1, number 1. Ohsawa intended to write forty-eight books for this series; he completed thirty-nine.*

The Unique Principle. George Ohsawa Macrobiotic Foundation, Oroville, California, 1978. Originally published as *Le Principe Unique de la Philosophie et de la Science d'Extrême Orient* by Librarie J. Vrin, Paris, 1931.

Vitamin C and Fruit. See *But I Love Fruits* on page 224.

You Are All Sanpaku. Award Books, New York, 1965. Attributed to Sakurazawa Nyoiti (George Ohsawa) but actually author William Dufty's reworking of texts by Ohsawa.

Zen Macrobiotics: The Philosophy of Oriental Medicine, Volume 1. The Ohsawa Foundation, Los Angeles, 1965. First published in English in mimeograph form by Ohsawa, New York, 1960, and in French as *Le Zen Macrobiotique* by Librarie J. Vrin, Paris, 1961.

ORIGINAL FRENCH TITLES

Acupuncture Macrobiotique (Macrobiotic Acupuncture). Sesam, Paris, 1961.

Aide–Mémoire de la Médecine Macrobiotique (A Small Guidebook of Macrobiotic Medicine). Chez L'Auteur, Paris, 1955.

Guide Pratique de la Médecine d'Extrême Orient. Chez L'Auteur, Paris, 1956.

Jack et Madame Mitie en Occident. See *Jack and Mitie in the West* in English Titles.

L'Acupuncture et la Médecine d'Extrême Orient. See *Acupuncture and the Philosophy of the Far East* in English Titles.

Le Cancer et la Philosophie d'Extrême Orient. See *Macrobiotics: The Way of Healing* in English Titles.

L'Ere Atomique et la Philosophie d'Extrême Orient. See *The Atomic Age and the Philosophy of the Far East* in English Titles.

Le Livre des Fleurs (The Book of Flowers). Librarie J. Vrin, Paris, 1931. Published in English in the *Macrobiotic Monthly, numbers 88, 89, 90, and 92,* in 1973.

Le Livre du Judo. See *The Art of Peace* in English Titles.

Le Philosophie de la Médecine d'Extrême Orient. See *Philosophy of Oriental Medicine* in English Titles.

Le Principe Unique de la Philosophie et de la Science d'Extrême Orient. See *The Unique Principle* in English Titles.

ORIGINAL JAPANESE TITLES
(titles listed in English; UP stands for Unique Principle Series)

Atomic Transmutation in Nature, with Louis Kervran. Publisher unavailable, Japan, 1963.

Biological Atomic Transmutation, with Louis Kervran. See *Biological Transmutations* in English Titles.

A Book of the Human Revolution. Publisher unavailable, Japan, 1948.

The Boys and Girls School for Health. Muso Genri Kokyujo, Ohtsu City, 1940.

Carrel's "Mankind": A Commentary. Principle Unique Center, Tokyo, 1947.

Challenge and Responses: Dr. Toynbee's Yin-Yang Principle. Publisher unavailable, Japan, 1946.

Clara Schumann. Konpa Shuppan Sha, Tokyo, 1948.

Compass. Monthly magazine from 1946 to 1956.

Compass Magazine Collections #3–#6. Nippon Center Ignoramus, Tokyo, 1960.

Concerning Proper Food. Publisher unavailable, Japan, 1941.

Correspondence Course of Natural Medicine #1. Publisher unavailable, Japan, 1938.

Correspondence to the Students at Maison Ignoramus. Monthly publication from 1957 to 1961.

Diet for Manchurian Life. Publisher unavailable, Japan, 1940.

Diet for Tuberculosis. Publisher unavailable, Japan 1936.

Dietetic Cure for Emphysema. Publisher unavailable, Japan, 1938.

Eternal Children: Anatole France and Romain Rolland. Muso Genri Kenkyujo, Ohtsu City, 1944. UP 5: 2.

The Eternal Youth: Biography of Benjamin Franklin. Publisher unavailable, Japan, 1952.

The Eternal Youth—Continued: Gandhi's Youth. See *Gandhi: The Eternal Youth* in English Titles.

The Ethics of Food and Eating. Nihon Shoku-Yo Kenkyujo, Ohtsu City, 1940.

Exploration of the Land of Bacteria. Muso Genri Kokyujo, Ohtsu City, 1943. UP III: 3–5.

The Final Event Man Will Face. Publisher unavailable, Japan, 1938.

The First Crossing of Equatorial Africa by a Japanese Woman, with Lima Ohsawa. Publisher unavailable, Japan, 1958.

Food and Human Life: A Guide for the "True Life" Movement. Publisher unavailable, Japan, 1943. UP II: 11–12.

Food Policy During Wartime (Correspondence Book #3). Publisher unavailable, Japan, 1941.

Foods for Thought. Publisher unavailable, Japan, 1938.

Foods for Victory in War. Dai Nihon Horei Shuppan, Tokyo, 1940.

Four-Thousand-Year History of China According to the Unique Principle. Muso Genri Kenkyujo, Ohtsu City, 1943. UP III: 1–2.

For My Students (Correspondence Book #4). Publisher unavailable, Japan, 1941.

A Free Man of 1,200 Years Ago—Dengyo Daishi (Compass Magazine Collection #1). Publisher unavailable, Japan, 1959.

Guidebook for Household Food Cures. Shoku-Yo Kai, Tokyo, 1937.

Guidebook for the Macrobiotic Healing Diet. Publisher unavailable, Japan, 1939.

Guidebook for the Right Diet. Publisher unavailable, Japan, 1939.

The Guiding Principles of the Department of Welfare and the Fundamental Unique Principle. Publisher unavailable, Tokyo, 1937.

Healing Foods. Publisher unavailable, Japan, 1940.

Health and Happiness Through Food. Shoku-Yo Kai, Tokyo, 1939.

Health. Magazine published from 1949 to 1959.

Health Notebook. Shoku-Yo Kai, Tokyo, 1939.

How to Cure the Heart. Publisher unavailable, Japan, 1944. UP V: 2.

How to Cure Sickness and How to Cure the Sick Man. Publisher unavailable, Japan, 1966.

How to Make Healthy Desserts. Publisher unavailable, Japan, 1939.

Human Nutritional Science and Medicine for the Health of Man. Dai Nihon Horei Shuppan, Tokyo, 1939.

An Invitation to Health and Happiness. See *Macrobiotics: An Invitation to Health and Happiness* in English Titles.

The Key to Heaven. Publisher unavailable, Japan, 1947.

The Last and Eternal Winner. Muso Genri Kenkyujo, Ohtsu City, 1943. UP II: 9.

Legend of Lake Mashu. Publisher unavailable, Japan, 1960.

Macrobiotic Cooking. Publisher unavailable, Japan, 1942.

Macrobiotic Cooking, with Lima Ohsawa. Publisher unavailable, Japan, 1953.

The Magic Spectacles. Publisher unavailable, Japan, 1940.

The Main Course of the Degrading of National Health (Correspondence Book #2). Publisher unavailable, Japan, 1941.

Mountain Fishing and Mushroom Hunting (Compass Magazine Collection #2). Publisher unavailable, Japan, 1960.

Musubi. Magazine published monthly from 1935 to 1946.

My Will. Publisher unavailable, Japan, 1938.

Mysterious World. Publisher unavailable, Japan, 1941. UP I: 2.

Nature Medicine: An Overview of Food Treatments. Publisher unavailable, Japan, 1938.

The New Science of Nutrition. Muso Genri Kokyujo, Ohtsu City, 1942. UP II: 2–8.

A New Dietetic Cure. Publisher unavailable, Japan, 1939.

A New Study of the Seven Articles on Military Strategy. Publisher unavailable, Japan, 1943.

Nutrition, Cooking, and Eating Brown Rice. Dai Nippon Horei Shuppan, Tokyo, 1940.

The Order of Man. Publisher unavailable, Japan, 1941. UP I: 3.

The Order of the Universe. See English Titles.

Our Health Line is Bombed. Publisher unavailable, Japan, 1941. UP I: 6.

Pasteur on Trial. Muso Genri Kenkyujo, Ohtsu City, 1943. UP II: 10.

Phenomena of Life and the Environment. Publisher unavailable, Japan, 1942. UP II: 1.

The Physiology of the Japanese Spirit (magazine collection). Nihon Shoku-Yo Kenkyujo, Tokyo, 1927.

The Poison of Sugar and the Harm of Eating Meat. Dai Nihon Horei Shuppan, Tokyo, 1939.

Primitive Mentality and the Japanese Mentality. Muso Genri Kenkyujo, Ohtsu City, 1943. UP III: 6–12.

The Principle of "Body and Soil are One." Publisher unavailable, Japan, 1936.

The Principle of Peace and Freedom. Publisher unavailable, Japan, 1949.

The Public Welfare Movement in Manchuria, with Tamura, Okawa, and Matsuda. Shoku-Yo Kai, Tokyo, 1940.

Rebirth. Magazine published monthly from 1919 to 1925.

Recipes for Health for Manchurian Life. Publisher unavailable, Japan, 1940.

A Report on Fifty Years' Experience in the Education of the Will. Nippon Center Ignoramus, Tokyo, 1966.

Report of the Hospital Experience. Publisher unavailable, Japan, 1941. UP I: 5.

Sagen Ishizuka. Publisher unavailable, Japan, 1928.

School for Health. Muso Genri Kokyujo, Ohtsu City, 1941.

Seven Articles on Military Strategy. Publisher unavailable, Japan, 1943. UP IV: 1.

Seven Conditions of Health. Publisher unavailable, Japan, 1966.

The Seven Great Conditions of Health: Concerning Justice. Publisher unavailable, Japan, 1962.

Shinto as a Natural Medicine: The Physiology of the Norito. Shoku-Yo Kai, Tokyo, 1936.

The Shoku-Yo Battle Line: Diet for Wartime. Shoku-Yo Kai, Tokyo, 1938.

The Shoku-Yo Guidebook for Living: A Plan for a Human Lifetime. See *Macrobiotic Guidebook for Living* in English Titles.

A Shoku-Yo Guidebook for Manchuria. Atago Insatsu, Japan, 1939.

The Shoku-Yo Seminars: Discourse on Macrobiotics. Five volumes taken from lectures: *Introduction; Principles of Diet; Dietary Healing I; Dietary Healing II; Cooking for Healing.* Publisher unavailable, Japan, 1928.

The Six Conditions of Health. Publisher unavailable, Japan, 1938.

Solution to Food Problems in Wartime (Correspondence Book #1). Publisher unavailable, Japan, 1941.

Standing on the Front Line of the Health War. Muso Genri Kokyujo, Ohtsu City, 1941.

The Story of Flip: A Book Review. Konpa Shuppan Sha, Tokyo, 1949.

The Teacher: Collins, with Jiro Ogawa. Publisher unavailable, Japan, 1952.

The Technique of Curing Disease. Nippon Center Ignoramus, Tokyo, 1956.

The Termination of Natural Science, The Birth of a New Weltanschauung. Publisher unavailable, Japan, 1941. UP I: 8–12.

A Theory of Economics According to the Unique Principle: The World of Dreams and Passion. Muso Genri Kenkyujo, 1944. UP IV: 2.

Toward Health and Happiness. Publisher unavailable, Japan, 1948.

Tragedy of Scientific Culture and Oriental Philosophy. Publisher unavailable, Japan, 1965.

Unhappy People, with Michi Ogawa. Publisher unavailable, Japan, 1941.

Unique Principle (Correspondence Book #5). Publisher unavailable, Japan, 1942.

The Unique Principle: I-Ching—A Practical Dialectical Method. Publisher unavailable, Japan, 1936.

The Unique Principle of the Eel. Muso Genri Kokyujo, Ohtsu City, 1941. UP I: 7.

Urination of the Rabbit. Publisher unavailable, Japan, 1941. UP I: 4.

Who Are Those Who Destroy Japan? Nihon Shuppan Haikyu Kabushiki, Tokyo, 1937.

Why Japan Must Fight With the White Race (No Reason). Publisher unavailable, Japan, 1932.

Why Was Japan Defeated? Muso Genri Kenkyujo, Ohtsu City, 1947. UP VI: 1.

World Government. Newspaper published from 1948 to 1959.

The World Journey of the Penniless Samurai. Institut de Philosophie et Médecine D'Extrême Orient, Paris, 1957.

INDEX